The Intermittent Fasting Cookbook

A Complete Guide for Weight Loss and Healthy Diet for Beginners Using 16/8 Intermittent Fasting Plus over 100 Meal Prep Recipes.

BY

Adele Tyler

All trademarks and brands within this book are for clarifying purposes only and are the owned by the owners themselves, not affiliated with this document.

Table of Contents

CHAPTER 5: SNACKS RECIPES FOR INTERMITTENT FASTING 116

Introduction

Intermittent fasting is an eating pattern in which we eat and fast with a gap of some hours with an aim to get some health benefits related to weight loss and better eating habits. It has numerous health benefits for everyone regardless of their gender and age. Yes, it is for all of you, including men, women, elders above 50s in their age, and even athletes.

There are many methods to perform intermittent fasting:

- 5:2 practice or two days fasting in a week

- Fasting on alternative days

- Time-restricted fasting or 16:8 intermittent fasting

- Fasting for 24 hours of fasting, eating and fasting method

From these fasting types, the 16:8 fasting is gaining popularity because of its amazing effects on weight loss. 16:8 intermittent fasting is convenient, safe, and feasible. You can begin by developing an eight-hour frame and restricting your food consumption to that length of time. Many people like to consume food between noon and 8 o'clock at night, as it means that you will only have to fast overnight and miss breakfast, and you can have a good lunch and dinner meal with some snacks during the day. That is why this window of eating and fasting is widely popular but there are other variations of having an eating and fasting window of your choice.

Reducing your consumption to several hours per day helps to reduce calories for the day.

The best aspect of intermittent fasting is that it useful in:

- Losing excess body fat

- Correcting hormonal imbalances

- Enhancing insulin sensitivity

- Improving cardiovascular health

- Improving mental awareness

- Regularizing sleep patterns

As one has a restricted time for eating, it is compulsory to take all the essential nutrients required by the body. There are different ways to follow the 16:8 fasting method. You can have your breakfast and start fasting from 3 p.m. In this type of Intermittent Fasting, you can have the combo of two meals that are breakfast and snack and start fasting from 3.p.m. Many recipes have been given in this book that are easy to prepare and can satisfy your taste buds so that you can enjoy this intermittent fasting period. For instance, you can eat Avocado Ricotta Energy Toast in breakfast, and Peanut Butter Jelly Apple Nachos in snacks and then start your fasting at 3 o'clock. You can follow the brunch and early dinner type of intermittent fasting. For instance, you can eat Roasted Veggie Quinoa bowl in the brunch and Chicken Enchilada Bowl in the dinner. Those who can skip breakfast and brunch; they can have lunch and late dinner type of intermittent fasting regime. They can eat Sweet Potatoes, Chickpeas, and Spinach Currsy in their lunch and Garlic Butter Brazilian Steak in dinner.

Any 16:8 intermittent fasting regime that you follow, recipes made with veggies, nuts, lean meat, and fruits will fulfill your diet and health requirements along with your weight loss. You will have a better and healthy lifestyle after shedding your extra pounds and improving your mental health.

Chapter 1: Basics of Intermittent Fasting

People have executed fasting for thousands of years, and it is the pillar of various religions and cultures across the globe. Today, modern types of fasting have brought the ancient tradition a new twist. 16:8 type of Intermittent Fasting is one of the most common fasting forms. Intermittent Fasting includes alternating between fasting and eating periods and has recently got quite common. Let me clear to you that fasting and starvation are different things. Starvation is an involuntary action due to lack of food, whereas, in fasting, we voluntarily avoid food for health or spiritual reasons. Let us dive into the amazing and interesting world of Intermittent Fasting.

1.1 Getting Started with Intermittent Fasting Regime

Intermittent Fasting is an eating pattern; it is not a diet. It is a way to organize your meals so that you get the most out of your food. Intermittent Fasting is not changing what you are eating, rather it is changing when you are eating it. It is the best way to get slim without being on an insane diet or reducing calories to nil. Most people consume larger meals in a shorter period. In reality, most of the time, you are going to try to maintain your calories in the same way as you begin fasting intermittently. Also, Intermittent Fasting is a healthy way of keeping muscle strength when getting lean.

Along with that, the key reason people attempt to fast intermittently is to lose weight. Shortly, we will discuss how Intermittent Fasting contributes to fat loss. Most importantly, Intermittent Fasting is among the best ways we have to take a lousy weight off while holding healthy weight on, as it needs very little behavioral change.

It is a very positive development, as Intermittent Fasting meets the definition of "simple enough that you are going to do it, but significant enough that it makes a difference."

To know how Intermittent Fasting contributes to fat loss, we must first recognize the distinction between the fed state and the fasted state. Your body is in a fed state when it digests and absorbs food. Usually, the fed state starts when you start eating and continue eating for three to five hours as your body digests and retains the food you have just eaten. When you are in a fed condition, it is very difficult for your body to burn calories because your insulin levels rise.

At that stage, your body is moving to what is recognized as the post-absorptive condition. It is only a fancy way to suggest that your body does not process a meal. The post-absorptive phase lasts for 8 to 12 hours after your last meal when you reach the fasted period. It is much simpler for your body to burn calories in a fast-paced condition because your insulin levels are low. If you are in a state of fast, your body will burn fat that has been inaccessible in a fed state. Since we are not in a fasted state until 12 hours after our last feeding, it is unusual for our bodies to be in this fat-burning condition. It is among the main reasons why people do Intermittent Fasting and lose weight without changing what they eat, how often they sleep, or how much they exercise. Fasting puts a person in a fat-burning condition that he/she seldom does during regular feeding.

1.2 Different Methods of Intermittent Fasting

There are various types of Intermittent Fasting. Schemes differ in the number of fasting days and calorie limits. Intermittent Fasting requires wholly or partly refraining from food for a certain period before eating normally again.

It is suggested by the proponents of this type of diet that it can offer weight-loss, improved fitness, and longer lifespans. Proponents of this diet contend that an Intermittent Fasting regimen is more straightforward to manage than conventional calorie-controlled meals. Each individual's experience of Intermittent Fasting is different, and different ways are suitable for different people. There are numerous ways of Intermittent Fasting, and people may choose any of them according to their choice. Keep reading to find out about different ways of doing Intermittent Fasting.

Type 1: Fasting 12 hours in a Day

The guidelines for this diet are straightforward. An individual is required to determine and stick to a 12-hour fasting period every day. According to several researchers, fast for 10–16 hours may cause the body to transform its stored fat into energy that moves ketones into the bloodstream. Its purpose is to promote weight loss. This form of Intermittent Fasting program can be an excellent opportunity for beginners. That is because the fasting duration is relatively short, a lot of fasting happens during sleep, and a person can eat the same number of calories every day. The best way to do the 12-hour fast is to include the time of sleep or rest in the fasting time frame. For instance, someone may select to fast between 7 p.m. to 7 a.m. in the next morning. He would need to end his dinner before 7 p.m. Then he would wait till 7 a.m. To eat breakfast, he can sleep for a lot of time in between.

Type 2: 16:8 Fasting

Fasting for 16 hours a day, excluding an 8-hour meal period, is called the 16:8 approach or the Lean gains method. In the 16:8 diet, men fast for 16 hours a day, and women fast for 14 hours. This form of Intermittent Fasting can be beneficial for someone who has already attempted 12-hour fast but has not seen any benefits.

Usually, people finish the evening meal at 8 p.m. in this type of fasting and then miss breakfast the next day. They do not eat until noon. Research on mice showed that restricting the feeding period to 8 hours saved them from Diabetes, Obesity, Inflammation, and Liver disease, even though they consumed the same total amount of calories as they consumed whenever they liked.

Type 3: Fasting Two Days a Week

People on a diet 5:2 eat normal quantities of nutritious food for five days and reduce calorie consumption for two days. For two fasting days, men typically eat 600 calories and women 500 calories. Generally, in a week, people split their fasting days. For instance, they can fast on Mondays and Thursdays and normally eat in the next few days of the week. There should be at least one non-fast day on days of fasting. There is minimal work on the 5:2 diet, also known as the Easy Diet. A study examined 107 obese or overweight women concluded that reducing calories twice weekly and constant calorie reductions resulted in equal weight loss. The study also showed that this diet lowered insulin levels and enhanced insulin sensitivity between participants. Small-level research examined the impact of this fast style on 23 fat women. In the span of one menstrual cycle, women lost 4.8 percent of their weight and 8.0 percent of their fat accumulation. Although, these proportions returned to normal for most women after five days of a regular diet.

Type 4: Fasting on Alternative Days

There are some differences in the alternative fasting day program, which includes fasting every other day. For certain people, alternate-day fasting mainly means avoiding solids on fasting days, whereas others take up to 500 calories. On the days of eating, people want to eat as often as they want.

One research shows that alternate-day fasting is beneficial for weight loss and heart safety in overweight adults. The researchers discovered that 32 individuals had lost 5.2 kilograms (kg) or just about 11 pounds over 12 weeks. Alternate-day fasting is an extreme version of Intermittent Fasting, and may not be appropriate for newcomers or those with an unhealthy life status. People should return to standard eating patterns on a non-fast day. Eating in this way decreases the overall calorie intake of a person, but does not restrict the particular foods that the individual consumes.

Type 5: 24-Hour Fasting Weekly

Fasting absolutely for 1 or 2 days each week, known as the Consume-Stop-Consume Diet, means eating no food 24 hours a day. A lot of people fast from breakfast to breakfast or lunch to lunch. Those on this diet plan can have coffee, tea, and other calorie-free beverages during fasting time. A 24-hour fast can be difficult and can lead to headaches, fatigue, or irritability. Many people notice that these symptoms become less severe over time as the body shifts to this new pattern. People have benefited from trying 12-hour or 16-hour fast before moving to 24-hour fast. People can return to regular eating habits on a non-fast day. Eating in this way decreases the overall calorie intake of a person, but does not restrict the specific foods that the individual consumes.

Type 6: Meal Skipping

This balanced approach to Intermittent Fasting can be great for starters. Occasionally, it means skipping meals. People will determine which food to miss according to their level of hunger or time constraints.

However, it is essential to consume healthy foods in every meal. Meal skipping is highly effective if individuals track and respond to their body's hunger signals.

People following this form of Intermittent Fasting will eat when they are hungry and miss meals when they are not. For some people, this may feel more natural than other fasting methods.

Type 7: The Warrior Diet

The Warrior Diet is a comparatively severe form of Intermittent Fasting. The Warrior Diet includes consuming very little, generally only a few portions of organic fruit and vegetables, over a 20-hour fasting period, and consuming a big meal at night. The food frame is usually only about 4 hours away. This kind of fasting could be best for people who have already tried other forms of Intermittent Fasting. Followers of the Warrior Diet claim that human beings are natural night time eaters and that snacking at night allows the body to develop nutrients in line with its circadian rhythms. During the 4-hour meal phase, people can make sure that they eat lots of tasty vegetables, meats, and healthy fats. They can also include some carbohydrates. Though it is possible to consume some foods during the fasting period, it may be difficult to adhere to strict rules about when and what to consume in the long term. Also, some people are struggling to eat such a big meal, before bedtime.

1.3 Benefits of Intermittent Fasting

The most apparent advantage of Intermittent Fasting is weight loss. Furthermore, there are several possible benefits beyond that, some of which were recognized since prehistoric times. Fasting durations were often referred to as 'purifications,' 'detoxifications' or 'cleanse,' but the idea is the same as to refrain from eating food for a specific time. People assumed that this duration of food withdrawal would clear up and reinvigorate their toxin systems.

Intermittent Fasting's Benefits to Women

Intermittent Fasting not only advantages one's waistline and chip off the excess weight but may also reduce the chances of developing various chronic diseases.

- o **Heart Health**

Heart disease has become a significant cause of death in the world. Hypertension, elevated LDL Cholesterol, and Triglyceride levels are some of the main dangers of developing heart disease. LDL cholesterol refers to Low Density Lipoproteins which is also referred as Bad Cholesterol as its increased level can accumulate cholesterol in the arteries leading to heart trouble. One research in 16 obese women found that Intermittent Fasting reduced blood pressure by six percent in just eight weeks. That study also searched that Intermittent Fasting reduced Triglyceride levels by 32 percent and LDL Cholesterol by 25 percent. However, there is no clear correlation between Intermittent Fasting and improved LDL Cholesterol and Triglyceride rates. Research in 40 normal-weight people showed that one month of Intermittent Fasting during the Islamic month Ramadan did not end in a decrease in LDL Cholesterol or Triglycerides. Superior quality studies with more rigorous methods are required before researchers can adequately measure Intermittent Fasting on heart safety.

- o **Diabetes**

Intermittent Fasting can also help to control and lower the chances of Diabetes effectively. Just like the constant calorie limits, Intermittent Fasting tends to minimize several of the diabetes complications. It is primarily done by lowering insulin levels and raising insulin resistance. In a randomized trial of more than 100 overweight individuals, six months of fasting lowers insulin resistance by 19 percent, and insulin rates by 29 percent.

The amount of blood sugar stayed the same. Also, it was shown that eight to twelve weeks of Intermittent Fasting decreased insulin levels by twenty-one to thirty percent and blood sugar levels by three to six percent in pre-diabetes patients. It is a state in which glucose levels are high but not elevated enough to help diagnose. Intermittent Fasting is not as helpful to women as it is to men in terms of blood sugar. A recent study suggests that blood sugar control deteriorated in women after 22 days of alternate-day fasting, even though there was no adverse effect on men's blood sugar. Given this risk factor, the decrease in insulin and insulin tolerance is likely to decrease the risk of diabetes, especially in pre-Diabetes patients.

  o **Weight Loss**

Intermittent Fasting could be an easy and efficient way to lose weight if done correctly, as daily short-term fasting will enable you to eat fewer calories and waste your pounds. Several reports indicate that Intermittent Fasting is as successful as conventional calorie-restricted diets for short-term weight loss. A research study in adults with obesity showed that Intermittent Fasting resulted in an average decrease of 15 lbs. over 3–12 months.

Another study found that Intermittent Fasting decreased body weight by 3–8% in overweight adults over 3–24 weeks. The study also found that participants decreased their waist size by 3–7 percent during the same time. It should be remembered that the long-term effects of Intermittent Fasting on women's weight loss remain. In the short-term effects, Intermittent Fasting tends to assist with weight loss. However, the amount you lose is likely to rely on the calorie count you consume during non-fast periods and how long you stick to this lifestyle.

o **It Helps You Eat Less**

Shifting to Intermittent Fasting can naturally help you to eat less. One research found that young people ate 650 calories less per day when their food consumption was limited to four hours. Another investigation in 24 healthy men and women looked at the impact of prolonged, 36-hour fast-eating patterns. Instead of consuming extra calories on the post-fasting day, the overall calorie balance of the people involved decreased significantly by 1,900 calories.

Health Benefits of Intermittent Fasting to Athletes

The growth hormone promotes development. This hormone enhances the immune system. It builds muscle, cartilage, and tendons. Children swim in the water, and they heal like Superman because of the benefits of it. Older adults who maintain it, will experience better wound healing and exercise rehabilitation. The growth hormone can be injected as a drug by the athletes for gaining strength, which is the reason it is a prohibited product in professional athletes. In that situation, natural ways to improve growth hormone secretion can be useful to athletes of all kinds.

o **Enhanced Flexibility**

Metabolic flexibility is the simplicity by which a person can move along energy sources from carbohydrates to fat and back again. Sustaining metabolic flexibility is an effective way to lead a healthier life for the average person interested in fitness and longevity. Metabolic flexibility is necessary for an athlete involved in success, fitness, and durability.

o **Decreased Inflammation**

To achieve the strength levels, an athlete must induce significant inflammation from the workout and then return from the inflammation. You require inflammation, but you do need inflammation to go down.

Each part of the coin is essential. All fasting does is boost your innate ability to lessen your inflammation. You get a major immune reaction from a hard workout. It is the point when a fasted exercise can show effects. When you are in the phase of fast, you are in a condition of very low inflammation. Then you start the workout, and inflammation goes towards the peak. It is a great response, and you should adhere to it.

o **Maintenance of Energy Utilization**

Chronic Calorie Restriction means death for an athlete. They are in dire need of power. They have to use their energy if they need it. Fortunately, research shows that Intermittent Fasting is one way to "decrease calories" without reducing energy.

Intermittent Fasting's Benefits to Adults

o **Enhanced Autophagy**

It is a great way for the cells to "eat themselves" and get rid of harmful cells and produce more active components. Without such a process, the chances of developing cancer increase as the damaged cells continue to multiply.

o **Circadian Rhythm**

Your internal body clock controls almost every cycle in your body, and a cluster of adverse impacts will occur when it is interrupted. You can reinstall your circadian clock when you take a little break from eating.

o **Improved Brain and Heart Functioning**

Your mind will perform in improved way and increase your ability to observe and learn.

Chapter 2: 16:8 Intermittent Fasting Protocol for Weight Loss

Part-day fasting, alternatively known as time-limited feeding or 16:8, is the user-friendly and maintainable method of Intermittent Fasting. Simply put, you fast over a certain number of, i.e., 16 hours every day, and then implement your regular diet for the rest of the day (eight hours). This method is prevalent as you do not need to count calories, monitor your meal sizes, feel hungry or limited, or skip out on social events. Among all fasting methods, the 16:8 implementation rate has increased in trend. That is the way people get prepared to adhere to in the longer term. Just when you are fasting and eating a part-day fasting day, it is up to you. You can select an eight-hour window that is best suited for you to consume in or, maybe, more importantly, use a 16-hour frame of time that is convenient for you to fast in.

2.1 Fundamentals of 16:8 Intermittent Fasting and its Working Principle

16:8 type of Intermittent Fasting means restricting the intake of food and calorie-containing drinks to a fixed time of eight hours a day and avoiding eating for the next 16 hours. You can perform this fasting as much as you like from one or two days of a week to each day of the week, based on individual preference. In recent years, Intermittent Fasting increased in popularity, particularly in those seeking to lose extra pounds of fat. Whereas other dieting plans lay down strict rules, 16:8 Intermittent Fasting is simple to implement and can deliver performance with a little effort.

It is usually considered less burdensome and more adaptable than various other dieting regimes and can fit easily into almost any way of living.

Moreover, to increase the process of weight loss, 16:8 Intermittent Fasting is often thought to boost blood sugar management. It also enhances brain activity and increases lifespan.

- **Starting a 16:8 Intermittent Fasting Regime**

16:8 Intermittent Fasting is easy, safe, and feasible. Begin by developing an eight hours' frame and restrict your food consumption to that length of time. Many people like to consume food between noon and 8 o'clock at night, as it means that you will only have to fast overnight and miss breakfast, and you can have a good lunch and dinner meal with some snacks during the day. Some choose to eat from 9 a.m. to 5 p.m. duration, which gives you enough time for a balanced breakfast at 9 a.m., a regular lunch at noon, and a small snack or early dinner at 4 p.m. prior you start fasting. However, you can choose the timeframe that fits best with your routine. Also, to optimize your health benefits from eating, it is necessary to commit to healthy foods and liquids during your diet. Loading up nutrient-rich foods will make you narrow down your consumption and enable you to get the benefits that this diet has to bring.

- **Possible Variations of 16:8 Intermittent Fasting Regime**

Following the Intermittent Fasting Protocol, you can choose your own choice of Fasting time and in your specific Feasting time, which combos of meal you can eat.

o **Have Your Breakfast and Start Fasting from 3 p.m.**

In this type of Intermittent Fasting, one can have the combo of two meals that are breakfast and snack and start fasting from 3.p.m.

It is going to be perfect for people who depend on breakfast to start their day energetically, and for singles who do not need to eat dinner with a family or a spouse at set times. This option is also perfect for people with heavy workloads, who usually turn to a toast or a ready meal for dinner.

o **Brunch and Early Dinner**

In this variation of Intermittent Fasting one can have the combination of two meals that is Brunch and early dinner. In these meals, one can choose the food of one's choice. This option is excellent for those who can skip breakfast but cannot get through to lunch without eating. It is also perfect for people who can have a break in the middle of the morning or eat at their office, and parents who want to have dinner earlier with their children.

o **Fast till the Lunch Time and Have Your Dinner Late**

In this variation of Intermittent Fasting, one can have the combo meals of lunch and late dinner. It is perfect for persistent breakfast avoiders, as well as those who can comfortably wait till lunch without eating. It also fits those who run late to work and get pastries or less nutritious breakfast choices on the ride. It is lovely for the company or switch workers who prefer to have a meal late. In this time period, people can eat their snacks and meals at reasonable times. Eating routinely is important to avoid highs and dips in blood sugar and to prevent excessive starvation. Some people may have to think and find the best food frame and meal periods for their lifestyle according to their needs.

2.2 How Does 16:8 Intermittent Fasting Work for Weight Loss?

Reducing your consumption to several hours per day helps to reduce calories for the day, but researches also demonstrate that fasting can increase metabolism and increase weight loss. Fasting is similar to Ketosis. Ketosis is a state in which the body has a deficiency of carbs and that reduced carbs are not enough to be used to consume energy. Then the body burns fats of the body for energy gain that results in fat loss. For your body to be in ketosis, you will fast in some way by either not eating any food anyway or maintaining carbs reasonably low. If you are in ketosis, it means that your body breaks down fat for fuel. Intermittent Fasting tends to reduce the glucose reserves at a quicker rate, which makes the cycle of fat running faster. Numerous people who start ketogenic diets start fasting to reach ketosis more quickly. When one follows both Keto diet and intermittent fasting, gets tremendous health benefits.

There are several ways to speed up Intermittent Fasting, but the most popular form is the split of 16 to 8. Or, for simplicity, some might call it a 16:8 fasting method. In this fasting program, you are going to keep fast for 16 hours straight a day and eat in the remaining 8-hour window. It may be tough to go without food for a long time at first, but it is something you can just be used to. And if you distribute the 16 hours wisely, it will be less hard to handle the fasting time.

For instance, if you use 8 hours of sleep in your 16-hour fasting, that is half of your fasting time. And simply saying, there is a lot of turnover between dinner and bedtime too. And that allows you an additional 3-4 hours.

For making up the rest, you will be fasting in the morning till lunch for four hours besides keeping yourself hydrated. Now, you have got 16 straight hours of fasting from about 7 p.m. to 11 a.m. the next morning. You need 16 hours for your 16/8 method. There would be a time of change, in the beginning, no doubt. But be careful with yourself, though.

2.3 Best Foods and Drinks to Break Intermittent Fast

Although you can eat from the food choices of your own, it is always better to have healthy food items which do not have a lot of fatty or sugary foods and drinks. Avoid eating processed or fast food and cut down excessive carbs. Include balanced food from all food groups including Carbohydrates, Protein, lots of vegetables, fruits, dairy, healthy fats and nuts with increased water intake.

- **Foods to Eat During Intermittent Fasting**

Calories always matter so; you can get as much nutrition as you can from any calories you consume. Mainly, during Intermittent Fasting phase, you should eat a specific type of healthy food that you might eat on almost any balanced diet. It means eating a lot of greens, lean protein, good fats, fish, whole grains, milk, and legumes. As these food groups hold the button to your Intermittent Fasting success, some decisions are even better than others if you make them according to your own food choices.

o **Vegetables**

Utilize a ton of green vegetables such as cauliflower, broccoli, and Brussel sprouts into your meal. They have got more fiber to help metabolism, and they are even helpful in making you feel fuller.

o **Legumes and Beans**

Chickpeas, black beans, and peas are useful for improving your strength, and they are also a great source of protein.

o **Fruits**

You would like to stop overloading the fruit because it includes a lot of natural sugar that disrupts insulin levels. Berries are a better option because of their high content of nutrients and antioxidants. Introducing berries and grains to the salads will enable you to have a variety of foods in one tasty serving.

o **Nuts**

Nuts have a small deal of fat and a variety of antioxidants. Although they are nutritious, they are also high in fat. Almonds, hazelnuts, walnuts, and cashews are a good option but in limited quantity.

o **Protein**

Lean beef, fish, and chicken are also healthy protein sources. Eggs are also a valuable source, and they are fast and easy to prepare. Getting more protein helps to fulfill the craving longer. It also enables you to develop the muscle you need to improve your metabolism.

o **Seafood**

Seafood is full of nutrients, particularly Omega-3 fatty acids. People who typically eat more Omega-3s reduce their risk of heart disease, depression, and anxiety. Shrimp, trout, and salmon are some of the better nutritionally-dense options.

o **Whole Grains**

Whole grains are also a great source of protein that is also abundant in fiber.

Choose whole grains, including rice and bread. Also, find some different foods like sorghum, Kamut, or spelt, and maybe you will find something that suits your palate and your new style of eating.

- **What to Drink During 16:8 Intermittent Fasting?**

o **Water**

It does not sound strange that you must drink lots of water and keep you hydrated throughout both Intermittent Fasting stages. And you are not limited to drinking water. You can also get zero-calorie drinks in the fasting and feeding slots. Sugar substitutes in diet sodas can, however, cause sugar cravings and reduce the likelihood of losing weight.

o **Bone Broth**

Bone broth is abundant in nutrients such as Calcium, Potassium, and essential minerals, and also Collagen, which is necessary for the skin, bones, and hair. Bone broth is a liquid that has been shown to enhance the safety of the joints and to replenish the electrolytes that are helpful over a longer period.

o **Black Coffee**

Coffee can help to reduce appetite during a fast but the point is that you will have to use it without sugar or cream if you really wish to lose weight. You can add sweeteners and a splash of milk, but be sure to keep your consumption below 50 calories.

o **Herbal Teas**

Much like other liquids, decaffeinated tea is a perfect way to remain hydrated and can also help to reduce your appetite. Make sure to drink pure, no sugar or less sugar, at least when you are fasting.

All we discussed so far was an introduction to Intermittent Fasting. We talked about how one can start Intermittent Fasting to get rid of undesired fat and unhealthy lifestyle. The benefits that have been mentioned in this book are of utmost significance for athletes, elders, and women. For enjoying a healthy and productive life, you can enjoy your eating with some pause. Now you are familiar with the basics of Intermittent Fasting and possible variations mentioned above. It is time to share some delicious recipes for breakfast, brunch, lunch and dinner, that you can try according to the variation you choose and the combo you want to eat during your Intermittent Fasting phase. You can try recipes and keep reading to avail of this blasting opportunity.

Chapter 3: Breakfast and Brunch Recipes for Intermittent Fasting

3.1 Tasty Breakfast and Brunch Recipes

Recipe 1: Avocado Ricotta Energy Toast

o Total Time: 5 minutes

o Serves: 1

Ingredients

- Whole-grain bread one slice
- Ricotta 2 tbsp.
- Mashed avocado ¼ ripe
- Flaky sea salt pinch
- Crushed flakes of red pepper one pinch

Instructions

Toast the bread. Put avocado, crushed red pepper flakes, ricotta, and sea salt. You can take it with hard-boiled eggs or scrambled eggs and a serving of fruit or yogurt.

Nutrition

- ✓ Energy: 288 calories
- ✓ Protein: 10 g
- ✓ Carbs: 29 g
- ✓ Fat: 17 g

Recipe 2: Chickpea Waffles in Greek Style

o Total Time: 30 minutes
o Serves: 2

Ingredients

- Chickpea flour ¾ cup
- Baking soda ½ tsp.

- Salt ½ tsp.
- ¾ cup of plain 2% Greek yogurt
- Large eggs 6
- Tomatoes, scallion, cucumbers, olive oil, yogurt, parsley, and lemon juice to serve
- Pepper and Salt

Instructions

1. Heat the oven to 200°F. On a rimmed baking sheet, put a wire rack and place it in the oven. Heat waffle iron according to the directions.

2. Mix the baking soda, flour, and salt in a big bowl. In a bowl, whisk the yogurt and eggs.

3. Mix the wet ingredients with the dry ingredients.

4. Coat the waffle iron lightly with a nonstick cooking spray. Layer 1/4 to 1/2 cup of the mixture in each segment of the iron and cook till it is golden brown, for four to five minutes. Switch the waffles to the oven and keep it warm. Repeat it for the remaining batter.

5. Offer waffles with a combination of savory tomatoes or a drizzle of hot almond butter and berries.

Nutrition

- ✓ Calorie 412
- ✓ Protein 35 g
- ✓ Carbs 24 g
- ✓ Fat 18 g

Recipe 3: Breakfast of Turkish Egg

- o Total Time: 13 minutes

- o Serves: 2

Ingredients

- Olive oil half tbs.

- Red bell pepper ¾ cup diced
- Eggplant ¾ cup diced
- Salt and pepper one pinch
- Lightly beaten Large eggs, 5
- Paprika ¼ tsp.
- Chopped Cilantro, to taste
- Plain yogurt two dollops
- Wheat pita one whole

Instructions

1. Place olive oil in a large nonstick skillet at medium height. Put bell pepper, eggplant, salt, and pepper. Simmer till softened, around seven minutes.

2. Mix in the eggs, paprika, and add salt and pepper to taste. Cook, frequently stirring, till the eggs are gently scrambled.

3. Sprinkle with chopped cilantro and serve with yogurt and pita.

Nutrition

- ✓ Calories 469
- ✓ Protein 25 g
- ✓ Carbs 26 g
- ✓ Fat 29 g

Recipe 4: Poached Eggs and Bacon on Toast

o Total Time: 20 minutes

o Serves: 1

Ingredients

- Bacon 2 slices

- Eggs 2 medium

- Salmon (If you want)

- Spinach baby leaf 200 grams
- Black pepper
- Sea salt
- Toast 1 slice

Instructions

1. Make a large pan of water to a gentle boil.
2. Stir the water gently and then break the eggs; poach for 4 minutes or until the whites are set.
3. During that time, heat a deep-frying pan, add a splash of water, and sprinkle with the spinach. Cook for 2 minutes until the mixture is withered.
4. Take spinach and place it aside on a plate. Fry the bacon till golden brown.
5. Put the spinach (and salmon) on a toast, sprinkle with salt and pepper.
6. Cover all of it with poached eggs and bacon.

Nutrition

- ✓ Calorie 270
- ✓ Carbs 3g
- ✓ Protein 26g
- ✓ Fats 21g

Recipe 5: Turmeric Tofu Scramble

o Total Time: 15 minutes

o Serves: 1

Ingredients

- Portobello mushroom 1
- Cherry tomatoes 3 or 4
- Tofu, firm ½ block

- Ground turmeric ¼ tsp
- Garlic powder one pinch
- Pepper and Salt
- Avocado ½ thinly sliced
- Olive oil, some more for brushing 1 tbsp.

Instructions

1. Make the oven to a temperature of 400 ° F. Put mushroom and tomatoes on a baking sheet and brush them with oil.

2. Sprinkle it with salt and pepper. Cook until tender, about ten minutes.

3. In the meantime, mix tofu, turmeric, garlic powder, and a pinch of salt in a medium dish.

4. Mash with a fork.

5. In a large electric frying pan, over medium heat, put 1 tbsp. of olive oil. Add the tofu mixture and cook stirringly, until solid.

Nutrition

- ✓ Calories 431
- ✓ Protein 21 g
- ✓ Carbs (8 g fiber) 17 g
- ✓ Fat 33 g

Recipe 6: Raspberry Jam and Peanut Butter Overnight Oats

- Total Time: 5 minutes
- Serves: 1

Ingredients

- Easy-cooking rolled oats ¼ cup
- 2 percent milk ½ cup
- Peanut butter, creamy 3 tbsp.
- Raspberries, (whole) 3 tbsp.

o   Raspberries mashed one-fourth cup

Instructions

1. In a medium bowl, combine oats, sugar, peanut butter, and squashed raspberries. Stir, until the batter is smooth.

2. Cover and chill overnight. In the morning, open and top with all the raspberries.

Nutrition

- ✓ Calories 328.5
- ✓ Fat 9.3g
- ✓ Protein 15g
- ✓ Carbs 48g

Recipe 7: Coconut Banana Bread

o   Total Time: 55 minutes

o   Serves: 6

Ingredients

- Small bananas 3 ripe
- Syrup of Rice malt 90 g
- Lightly whisked eggs 3 medium
- Bicarbonate of Soda, three fourth teaspoon
- Vanilla extract which is alcohol free, a few drop
- Salt, half teaspoon
- Coconut flour 30 g
- For serving, Fruit

Instructions

1. Settle the oven to 180 ° C and do the greasing of a tin of twenty-one into nine cm. bars.

2.   Please take off the peel of bananas and make a puree of them in a small bowl. Then put the eggs, vanilla, rice malt syrup, and combine.

3. Add bicarbonate soda, flour, and salt and whisk well. In a prepared tin, put the mixture.

4.   Then keep it for baking for 50 minutes or until the spatula in the center of the bread can come out clear. Cool entirely on a wire rack in a tin, then make a slice and present with fruit.

Nutrition

- ✓ Calories: 223
- ✓ Carbohydrates: 30g
- ✓ Protein: 3g
- ✓ Fat: 9g

Recipe 8: Almond Apple Spice Muffins

o Total Time: 15 minutes

o Serves: 5

Ingredients

- Butter, half stick
- Almond meal, 2 cups
- Eggs, 4 larges
- Unsweetened applesauce 1 cup
- Cinnamon 1 tbsp.
- Protein powder of Vanilla 4 scoops
- All spice 1 tsp
- Cloves 1 tsp.
- Baking powder 2 tsp

Instructions

1. Settle the oven to 350 degrees F. Melt the butter in the microwave at low heat for almost 30 seconds in a small microwave-secure bowl.
2. In a large tub, combine the rest of the ingredients thoroughly with the butter. Sprinkle two muffin tins with a nonstick cooking spray or using a cupcake lining.
3. Pour the mixture into the muffin tins, ensuring that it is not overfilled (about three-fourths full). We expect to prepare ten muffins.
4. Position a tray in the oven and bake for 12 minutes. Make sure you do not overcook because the muffins will be too hard. When it finishes, take out the first utensil from the oven and bake the second tin likewise.

Nutrition

- ✓ Calories 484
- ✓ Protein 40 g
- ✓ Carbs 16 g
- ✓ Fat 31 g

Recipe 9: Chewy Cinnamon Rolls

o Total Time: 70 minutes

o Serves: 15

Ingredients

For Rolls

- All-purpose flour 3 cups
- Whole-wheat flour 1 cup
- Dry yeast ¼ ounce(active)
- Sugar ¾ cup
- Milk plain/ soymilk 1 cup
- Vegetable oil ¼ cup

- Salt 1tsp
- Egg whites 4
- Margarine ¼ cup
- Cinnamon 2 teaspoons

For Glaze

- Half teaspoon pure vanilla extract
- Powdered sugar 1 cup
- Soymilk 2 tablespoons

Instructions

1. In a large mixing pot, add 1 cup of all-purpose flour, whole-wheat flour, and yeast. Set it aside.

2. Merge the soya milk, one-fourth cup of the sugar, oil, and salt in a large pan and heat until hot.

3. Whisk in the mixture, then add flour as well as the yeast mixture. Whisk the whites of the egg.

4. Pummel at high speed for around four minutes, periodically slowing to scratch down the sides.

5. To create a firm dough, whisk in the greater portion of the leftover all-purpose flour.

6. Start taking the dough from the mixer bowl and place it on a floured surface. Make the dough for around 10 minutes, then apply further flour to the tablespoon to keep it from binding.

6. Position the dough in a bowl that is greased with oil, and switch it over to the tip of the dough tub. Shield with a cloth and let it grow in a warm position till it doubles in size (about an hour).

7. Roll the risen dough and break it into two parts. Roll each piece of dough into a one-fourth inch thick rectangular shape.

8. Heat the margarine and dab it on the rectangle of the flour. Combine the cinnamon and the leftover half cup of sugar in a small container and scatter the mixture properly over both squares of the crust.

9. Roll up the rectangles, beginning with the most extensive edges. Press your fingers to close the ends and push the margins to the dough.

10. Form the rolls to 1inch pieces and place the portions cut sideways in two greased baking bowls or 9 inch round nonstick dishes. Cap each container with a cloth or waxed paper and allow the rolls to raise in a hot environment until they are doubled (about 45 minutes). Settle the oven to 375 degrees.

11. Bake for around 20 minutes.

12. When the rolls get baked, prepare the glaze by adding the vanilla, sugar, and tablespoon of the soya. Start adding soymilk by enhancing it with one teaspoon until the glaze is dense, but we can pour it. Sprinkle the glaze over the hot rolls and serve.

Nutrition

- ✓ Calories 535
- ✓ Carbohydrates 93g
- ✓ Protein 7g
- ✓ Fat 16g

Recipe 10: Roasted Broccoli with Lemon, Garlic and Toasted Pine Nuts

- o Total Time: 40 minutes
- o Serves: 2

Ingredients

- Broccoli 1 large head (one and half pounds), cut into stems and florets

- Freshly ground pepper
- Kosher salt
- Minced shallot 1 teaspoon
- Olive oil (extra-virgin) 1/4 cup
- Fresh lemon juice 2 teaspoons
- Pine nuts 1 1/2 tablespoons

Instructions

1. Settle the oven to 400 ° C. Place the broccoli flowers and stems on a wide baking sheet with two tbsp. of olive oil and sprinkle with salt.

2. Bake the broccoli in the oven for around 30 minutes, stirring halfway through, till tender and browned.

3. Meanwhile, in a small pan, roast the pine nuts on moderate flame unless golden for approximately four minutes.

3. In a small pan, combine the lemon juice with a shallot and the leftover 2 tablespoons of olive oil; sprinkle with salt and pepper. Spread the broccoli in a serving dish. Then put the toasted nuts of pine and dressing, garnish well and present.

Nutrition

- ✓ Calorie 172.7
- ✓ Fat 15.8 g
- ✓ Carbs 7 g
- ✓ Protein 4.1 g

Recipe 11: Hard Boiled Eggs

- o Total Time: 12 minutes
- o Serves: 6

Instructions

1. Put the eggs in a medium saucepan. Line with 1"of water over the eggs. Position a cooktop over high heat.

2. Wait for the eggs to a boil. Take off immediately from heat and put a cover. Wait for 18-20 minutes.

3. Put the cold water from the tap into the pan, letting the hot water drain away by keeping the bowl on an angle. Keep the eggs in cold water for one to two minutes, then peel easily.

Nutrition

- ✓ Calories 78
- ✓ Total fat 5.3 g
- ✓ Total carbs 0.6 g
- ✓ Protein 6.3 g

Recipe 12: Breakfast Tart

o   Total Time: 25 minutes

o   Serves: 4

Ingredients

- 1 cup of chopped nuts
- Coconut oil 1/4 cup
- Old fashioned oats one and a half cups
- Brown sugar 2 Tbsp.
- Vanilla extract 1 tsp

Filling and topping

- Vanilla 24 ounce
- Small star fruit, thinly sliced One large or two
- Strawberries sliced 2-3
- Mandarin /orange slices 1/2 cup
- Blueberries 1/2 cup
- Mango or papaya thinly sliced One
- Kiwi peeled and sliced One

- Banana 1/2

- about ten raspberries

Instructions

1. Set the oven at 350F

2. Combine the oats, seeds and nuts, coconut oil, sugar and vanilla together in a bowl until everything is well coated.

3. Push the mixture into a lubricated 10-12 inches' tart pan with a pie plate. Choose a measuring cup to support you pushing the granola uniformly around the pan and up the sides. You do not need all the mixture based on the pan.

4. Bake for around 15 minutes, until it is slightly golden. Let it chill. If you would like to, you could create the crust ahead and fill it in the next morning just before serving.

5. Layer the yogurt uniformly over the chilled granola surface.

6. Organize the strawberries optionally with the star fruit slices, starting at the outer edge. Add the mandarin orange slices in the areas between them.

7. After that, set down a circle of halved blueberries. Follow the hearts of the mango and the raspberries.

8. Organize half the kiwi moons after that, and fill the center with banana slices, blueberries and raspberries.

9. Serve immediately for best results. Remove the edges of the tart pan so that you can cut your tart more easily. Choose a sharp knife to cut through the dough and ease the pieces with the pie server.

Nutrition

- ✓ Calories 230
- ✓ Fat 16.6 g
- ✓ Protein 6.9 g
- ✓ Carbs 17.7 g

Recipe 13: Vegan Lentil Burger

- o Total Time: 2 hour and 10 minutes
- o Serves: 6

Ingredients

- Brown lentils 3/4 cup
- Extra-virgin olive oil 2 teaspoons
- Low-sodium vegetable broth or water 1and3/4 cups
- Red onion, half thinly sliced and half chopped 1 large
- Juice of half lemon
- Kosher salt
- Fresh spinach 8 ounces
- Garlic cloves, minced 2 large
- Black pepper
- Ground cumin, half teaspoon
- Whole-wheat bread crumbs 1 cup
- Cooking spray
- Walnuts, toasted and finely chopped half cup
- Whole-grain vegan buns 6

Instructions

1. Take the lentils and 1 3/4 cup of the broth for boiling on high temperature in a medium saucepan. Decrease heat to medium-low, partly covered, and cook until the lentils are entirely softened, and the liquid is absorbed for around 30 minutes.

2. Mix it with the leftover one tablespoon of the broth and mix well with the stick blender. Set it aside.

3. Warm the oil over the medium temperature in a large nonstick skillet. Add the lemon juice, chopped onion, and 1/4 teaspoon salt and cook for around 6 minutes, stirring till soft.

4. Add the spinach, garlic, 1 and a half teaspoons of black pepper and cumin, and stir until the spinach is withered for around 3 minutes.

3. Add the mixture of spinach, breadcrumbs, walnuts, and salt to the lentils and blend thoroughly. Put a cover and refrigerate for at least one hour or overnight.

4. Heat the grill to medium-high. Shape the mixture into six 4-inch patties and sprinkle each side with a cooking spray. Grill till pleasant grill marks are formed, around 3 minutes per hand. Put the patties in the buns with the chopped onion and other seasonings and eat.

Nutrition

- ✓ Calories 560
- ✓ Total Fat 14g
- ✓ Carbs 90 g
- ✓ Protein 21g

Recipe 14: Savory Oatmeal Bowl

- o Total Time: 20 minutes
- o Serves: 1

Ingredients

- Old fashioned oatmeal ½ cup
- 1 cup of water
- dash of sea salt
- One cooked egg
- 2 Tablespoons grated parmesan cheese
- 3–4 grape tomatoes
- 1/4 avocado
- Everything but The Bagel seasoning
- Sea salt and pepper
- Fresh herbs, for topping
- Hot sauce (optional)

Instructions

1. Heat the water and the oatmeal in a medium saucepan over lower temperatures.

2. Put a little sea salt in the oats. Prepare the oats, rolling periodically for 5-7 minutes or until the oats are smooth and the consistency you want.

2. In the meantime, cook your egg as much as you want, poached or fried is your preference.

3. When the oats and the eggs are cooked, take a bowl and put the oats and do the topping with cooked egg, avocado, parmesan cheese, everything but the bagel seasoning, fresh herbs, and hot sauce.

Nutrition

- ✓ Calories 330
- ✓ Fat 16g
- ✓ Carbohydrates 32g
- ✓ Fiber 7g
- ✓ Protein 16g

Recipe 15: Vegan Coconut Kefir Banana Muffins

- o   Total Time: 60 minutes
- o   Serves: 12

Ingredients

- All-purpose flour, one and a half cups
- Crushed sugar, 1 cup
- Unsweetened shredded coconut 250 mL
- Baking soda 2 teaspoon
- Baking powder 1 teaspoon
- Salt 1/2 tsp
- Ripe mashed bananas 2
- Coconut milk, dairy-free one and a half cups
- Pure Vanilla extract 1 tsp
- Liquid Coconut Oil, one-fourth cup

Instructions

1. Settle the oven to 180 ° C. Sprinkle cooking spray on muffin tin. Put it aside.

2. In a big bowl, whisk together sugar, flour, baking powder, shredded coconut, salt, and baking soda. Place it aside.

3. In a separate big cup, mix together bananas, vanilla, and coconut oil. Put the flour and mix, whisk until there are no white stripes left.

4. Add mixture in muffin pot. Keep baking till the upper parts are golden and the spatula put in the middle comes out clear, around 30 minutes. Allow chilling the muffin tin for 15 minutes.

Nutrition

- ✓ Calorie 212
- ✓ Total Fat 7g
- ✓ Carbs 35g
- ✓ Protein 2g

Recipe 16: Burrito Bowl with Chipotle Black Beans

- o Total Time: 30 minutes
- o Serves: 2

Ingredients

- Basmati rice 125g
- Garlic cloves, 2
- Cider vinegar 1 tbsp.
- Olive oil 1 tbsp.
- Black beans, rinsed 400g Tin
- Honey 1 tsp.
- Red onion, chopped 1 small
- Chipotle paste 1 tbsp.
- Chopped curly kale 100g
- Tomato, chopped 1 medium
- Avocado 1 sliced for serving (optional)
- Chipotle hot sauce
- Coriander
- Wedges of Lime

Instructions

1. Cook the rice, then rinse and transfer to the pan to keep it warm. Warm the oil in a frying pan, add garlic and cook for 2 minutes or till it is golden. Include the beans, honey, vinegar, and chipotle. Simmer and heat for 2 minutes.
2. Cook the kale for 1 min, drain and drop out any excess water. Split the rice into large shallow bowls and top with the beans, avocado, kale, tomato, and onion. Present with coriander, sauce, and lemon wedges, if you prefer.

Nutritional Value

- ✓ Calories 573
- ✓ Fat 21g
- ✓ Protein 16g
- ✓ Carbs 72g

Recipe 17: Trial Mix

- o Total Time: 15 minutes
- o Serves:

Ingredients

- Almonds, slightly salted and dry roasted 3 parts
- Raw walnuts 2 parts
- Cashews, dry-roasted & unsalted, 1 part
- Raw pecans 2 parts
- Dried cherries or cranberries, or fruit-juice sweetened 1 part
- Unsweetened flaked coconut 1 part
- Semi-sweet chocolate chips 1 part

Instructions

1. Add all the ingredients in a bowl.

2. Softly stir to mix.

3. Place it in an airtight jar.

Nutrition

- ✓ Calorie 183
- ✓ Carbs 9g
- ✓ Protein 4g
- ✓ Fat 16g
- ✓

Recipe 18: Teacup Watermelon Salad

- o Total Time:15 minutes
- o Serves:3

Ingredients

- Diced seedless watermelon 350 g
- Mint leaves, Chopped Small handful
- Baby English spinach leaves 90 g
- Red onion, thinly sliced 1 1/2
- Large celery stalk, thinly sliced
- Goat's cheese crumbled 60 g

For Dressing

- Lime juice, 1 tsp.
- Lime juice, 1 tsp.
- Sheep's milk yoghurt 130 g
- Freshly ground black pepper, as per taste and Celtic sea salt
- Coriander, chopped, Handful

Instructions

1. In a small utensil, whisk all the dressing ingredients together.

2. Add the ingredients of salad into a large bowl, split among three large- heaped teacups, mugs or bowls. Put the dressing on top and serve immediately.

A tip as a bonus:

Put the salad and dressing separately till just before serving, when you are ready to eat, pour the dressing spoon on top.

Nutrition

- ✓ Calories144
- ✓ Fat 5.6 g
- ✓ Carbs 15 g
- ✓ Protein 5.3 g

Recipe 19: Roasted Veggie Quinoa Bowl

o   Total Time: 30 minutes

o   Serves: 2

Ingredients

Broccoli (Garlic Roasted)

- 2 Cups of Broccoli
- 2 tsp of canola oil
- Black pepper
- Garlic, minced 2 cloves
- Salt, a pinch

Roasted Sriracha and Soy Sauce Chickpeas

- Chickpeas (cooked) 1.5 cups

- Olive oil 1 tsp.

- Soy sauce 2 tsp.

- Sriracha 2 tsp.

Curry Roasted Sweet Potatoes

- Olive or canola oil 1 tsp

- Sweet potato 1 small

- Curry powder 1 tsp.

- Sriracha 1 tsp.

- Salt, a pinch

Chili Lime kale

- Chopped kale 2 cups

- Oil 1 tsp.
- Lime juice 1/4 tbsp.
- Pepper, a pinch
- Chili powder 1/2 tsp
- One pinch of salt

Garlic Roasted Broccoli

- Broccoli 2 cups
- Garlic, minced 2 cloves
- Black pepper
- Olive or canola oil 2tsp.
- Pinch of salt

Quinoa

- Quinoa, rinsed ¾ cup
- Vegetable broth 1.5 cups

Optional

- Lime
- Red pepper flakes
- Hummus
- Guacamole
- Avocado

Instructions

1. Set 400F temperature of the oven. Cover a wide baking tray of parchment paper.

2. Prepare the vegetables: cut the broccoli into normal-sized balls, destem and cut the kale, clean and cut the sweet potato to 1/4-inch pieces.

3. Rub the broccoli flowers with garlic, oil, pepper, and salt. Be sure all the ingredients are in the upper surface of the flowers. Position them down the middle third of the large baking tray in a line.

4. Use the same bowl that you used to mix the broccoli, add the chickpeas, oil, soya sauce, and Sriracha. Be sure that you place them in a line alongside the broccoli.

5. In that same container, put the oil, curry powder, salt, and Sriracha. Put the chopped sweet potatoes and twist to coat. Place the rings on the left over one third of the baking sheet.

6. Bake for about 10 minutes. Turn the sweet potatoes and broccoli and again divide the chickpeas to facilitate further cooking. Toast for more eight to twelve minutes.

7. **For Quinoa:** Wash the quinoa and drain it. Place the washed vegetable broth, and quinoa in a small pan and wait for a boil over high flame. Switch the heat to moderate-low, put a cover, and seethe for approximately 15 minutes. After frying, fluff with a fork and set aside.

8. **Kale:** When the quinoa is boiling, and the rest of the ingredients are cooking, heat a large skillet with one teaspoon of oil. Add the kale and cook for almost five minutes, or almost before it is tender. Add oil, chili powder, lime juice. Toss to coat and cook for a further two to three minutes.

9. **For Serving:** Scoop one to two cups of quinoa in each dish, top with half broccoli, half chickpeas, half kale, and half sweet potatoes. Put everything in a bowl or to mix it all.

Nutrition
- ✓ Calories 415
- ✓ Carbs 54g
- ✓ Protein 16g
- ✓ Fat 17g

Recipe 20: Cinnamon Butter with Fig Toast

o Total Time: 5 minutes

o Serves: 8

Ingredients

- Cinnamon 1/2 teaspoon
- Blends plant-based butter Blends 1/4 cup
- Vanilla extract 1/4 teaspoon

- Cardamom 1/16 teaspoon
- Maple syrup 2 tablespoons

For Fig Toast

- Sourdough bread 8 slices
- Fresh figs, 8–10
- Roasted crushed pistachios
- Flaky Sea salt
- Finely cut Fresh mint

Instructions

1. In a sealed jar, mix together all the components for cinnamon butter. Savor and change the ingredients as you like. Put the cover on and place it in the refrigerator. You are able to use it now.

2. For the fig toast: Bake the bread till it is as crispy as you want it to be. Layer about half tablespoon of cinnamon butter around each slice of toast. Top with chopped figs, pistachio, mint and salt as required.

Nutrition

- ✓ Calories 322
- ✓ Fat 10g
- ✓ Carbs 40g
- ✓ Protein 16g

Recipe 21: Gingerbread Scones with Vanilla Bean Glaze
- o Total Time: 30 minutes
- o Serves: 6-8

Ingredients

- Whole wheat pastry flour 2 cups
- Coconut sugar ⅓ cup
- Baking powder 1 Tbsp.

- Cinnamon ½ tsp

- Sea salt ¼ tsp

- Coconut oil or vegan butter 5 Tbsp.

- Cloves ¼ tsp

- Flax egg 1

- Ginger 1 tsp

- Unsweetened almond milk ½ cup

- Molasses ⅓ cup

Glaze

- Vanilla bean ½

- Powdered sugar ¾ cup

- 1 Tbsp. of almond milk (unsweetened)

Instructions

1. Settle the oven to 400 degrees. Arrange a baking sheet of parchment paper.

2. Start to make your flax egg in a medium dish. Let it stay for 5 minutes.

3. First, add all your dry ingredients and stir in a large bowl.

4. After your flax egg has been sitting for 5 minutes, add the almond milk and the molasses. Stir to blend it fully. It takes a minute or two. Set it aside.

5. Add coconut oil to the dry ingredients. Split the coconut oil into the mixture using a pastry cutter or fork until the coconut oil is on the edge of the peas.

6. After that, carefully pour your wet ingredients in a dry place. Blend until it has just been mixed (careful not to overmix). There is still a little flour in the bottom of the bowl. That's all right!

7. Grab your scone batter and place it on the lined baking sheet. Shape into a circle of 7-8 inches.

8. Use a sturdy knife, cut into eight equal triangles.

9. Put it in the microwave and toast for about 14 minutes.

10. After 14 minutes, cut the scones again (where you cut them) and pull them apart so that the sides have time to bake.

11. Bake for 2-4 more minutes (16-18 minutes in total). Or till it is golden brown and cooked thoroughly.

12. Let it cool for 10 minutes.

13. Mix all the ingredients to a bowl and whisk to smoothen and to make the glaze. Sprinkle on the crest of your scones. Maintain scones completely covered for freshness.

Nutritional Value

- ✓ Calories 333
- ✓ Fat 11
- ✓ Carbs 54
- ✓ Protein 6

Recipe 22: Butternut Squash

- o Total Time: 50 minutes
- o Serves:4

Ingredients

- Butternut squash One large
- Olive oil 2–4 tablespoons
- Pepper
- Salt

Instructions

1. Initially, settle the oven to 400oF.

2. After that, utilize a vegetable peeler to scrape the butternut squash.

3. Use a honed knife to cut a half hot dog type butternut squash. Don't be scared to take a little muscle in it!

4. When cut in half, choose a spoon to eliminate any seeds and flesh from inside.

5. Then, cut that off! We want to chop a butternut squash into bite-sized pieces so that it can be cooked faster. Please ensure all the parts are cut to approximately the same size so that they are efficiently baked.

6. Sprinkle with olive oil and season with salt, pepper and any other spices that your heart desires.

7. Toss it with your fingertips, then place it in the oven.

8. Grill for 25-30 minutes, halfway tossed.

Nutrition

- ✓ Calories 153
- ✓ Fat 10
- ✓ Carbs 16
- ✓ Protein 1

Recipe 23: Iced Matcha Latte

o Total Time: 5 minutes

o Serves: 2

Ingredients

- One teaspoon of premium quality matcha powder

- 1/2 tablespoon Octane Oil

- 1/2 tsp. stevia powder (or preferred sweetener to taste)

- 1 tsp. of vanilla

- One tablespoon of collagen protein

- 150 g (or 1 cup) of coconut milk, frozen into ice cubes 1 cup of water

- 1/2 – 1 teaspoon of ashwagandha

Instructions

1. In a high-powered processor, add all ingredients except collagen content.

2. Batter until smooth and well-combined.

3. If possible, try and change the sweetness.

4. To avoid destroying proteins, add the collagen softly before it is even added.

5. Spoon over the ice and thoroughly enjoy it.

6. It is ready to serve one person.

Nutrition

- ✓ Calories 224
- ✓ Carbs 3g
- ✓ Fat 21g
- ✓ Protein 2g

Recipe 24: Fluffy Paleo Pancakes by Almond Flour

o Total Time: 20 minutes

o Serves: 4

Ingredients:

- Cinnamon one tsp.

- Marine salt 1/4 tsp.

- Baking soda 1/2 tsp.

- Big pastured eggs 3

- Almond flour 1 1/2 cups

- Take 1/4 cup pasture coconut milk that is kept at room temperature.

- Vinegar apple cider 1/4 tsp.

- Unsalted butter 1 tbsp.
- Liquid stevia 1/8t tsp.
- Vanilla extract 2 tsp.

Instructions

1. Preheat the grid over medium flame.

2. Place the ingredients in liquid form in your blender and cover with all the dry components. Cover and mix to start at low, then rise to more speed and mix at least one full minute.

3. Grease butter panel which should be preheated.

4. Put a full spoon of flour onto the grid to create a pancake (approximately 3 inch in diameter) of silver dollars.

5. Flip as long as the batter begins bubbling Repeat until the mixture is done

Nutrition

- ✓ Calories 261
- ✓ Fat 23g
- ✓ Protein 9g
- ✓ Carbs 4g

Recipe 25: (Cannabidiol) CBD Rooibos Tea Latte

- o Total Time: 6 minutes
- o Serves: 1

Ingredients:

- 1 cup water and two bags rooibos tea
- One tablespoon grass-fed butter, or 1/4 cup full-fat coconut condensed milk (free of BPA)

- One teaspoon Brain Octane
- One scoop collagen peptide
- One dropper maximum CBD oil
- Optional: liquid monk fruit extract to taste, Ceylon cinnamon powder

Instructions

1. Boil water; add both tea bags to a cup, and for 5 minutes' steep.
2. Remove the tea bags and add the remaining ingredients except for collagen
3. Pour the mixture into a mixer and blend until it is mixed. To avoid damaging fragile proteins, add collagen, and mix at the lowest level until just combined.
4. Enjoy hot or pour ice over it.

Nutritional Value

- ✓ Calories 132
- ✓ Fat 11g
- ✓ Carbs 2g
- ✓ Protein 10g

Recipe 26: Veggie Keto Scramble

o Total Time: 20 minutes

o Serves: 1

Ingredients:

- Butter One cup
- Mushrooms   1 oz.
- Three eggs 1 oz. cut.
- Red bell peppers,
- Black pepper 1 oz. diced salt and field.

- Parmesan cheese   1/2 scallion sliced and diced

Instructions

1. Heat the butter over medium flame in a large frying pan. Put the sliced mushrooms, diced red peppers, salt, and fry until tender.

2. Add eggs directly into the pan and then mix so that all is well blended.

3. Keep moving the spatula to form large, soft curds across the bottom and side of the skillet.

4. Cook until the egg is clear, but the eggs are not complete.

5. Put the scramble with shredded parmesan and scallions on a plate on the tip.

Nutrition

- ✓ Carbs 4 g
- ✓ Fat 31 g
- ✓ Protein 28 g

Recipe 27: Classic Bacon and Eggs

o   Total Time: 15 minutes

o   Serves: 4

Ingredients:

- Eight eggs
- Slices of bacon 5 oz.
- Cherry tomatoes (optional)
- Fresh parsley (optional)

Instructions

1. In a medium-high heat pan, fry the bacon until crispy. Put on a plate away. Leave the fat in the pot.
2. For frying the eggs, use the same plate. Layer the eggs in the bacon grease over medium heat. You can also mix

them into a measuring cup and brush gently into the pan to avoid hot grease splattering.

3. Cook the eggs whatever way you like. For a sunny side up, put the eggs on one side to scramble and put the lid on the pan to make sure they are cooked up. Cooked over quick for eggs, roll over the eggs after a couple of minutes and cook for another minute. Split in half the cherry tomatoes and immediately fry them.

4. To try the salt and the pepper.

Nutrition

- ✓ Calories: 272kcal
- ✓ Net carbs: 2% (1 g)
- ✓ Fiber: 0 g
- ✓ Fat: 22 g
- ✓ Protein: 15 g

Recipe 28: Coconut Flour Crepe

o Total Time: 20 minutes

o Serves: 8-10

Ingredients

- Extra virgin coconut oil melted, 1 tbsp.
- Almond milk or water 1/4 cup
- Coconut cream melted 1/4 cup
- Eggs 4
- Vanilla extract 1/2 tbsp.
- Coconut flour 2 tbsp.
- Almond meal often known as almond flour 1 tbsp.

Instructions

1. Place all the components in a large mixing bowl: eggs, almond milk, extra virgin coconut oil, vanilla extract, coconut cream, and coconut meal

2. Beat up to an even batter, with no chunk using a whisk or electric mixer. Set aside to let the coconut flour to immerse the liquid for 10 minutes and stiffen the batter slightly.

3. Steam a medium/high heat slightly oil small pan. Utilize coconut oil with a sheet of tissue paper and brush on the plate. Use a pan of 4.7-inch. For making perfect crepes that do not break, I suggest a small saucepan of this type.

4. Pour the one-fourth cup of crepe batter on a pan, then point and gently tilt the pan to scatter the batter as lightly as you can. First brown, on the one hand, cook around two to three minutes until the surfaces become crispy and quickly pop out of the oven. Once you turn over, the middle should be placed and dry to keep the crepe from cracking.

5. Make them brown between one to two minutes on other sides and present hot with your preferred fillings.

Nutrition

- ✓ Calories 108
- ✓ Fat 8.9g
- ✓ Carbohydrates 2.5g
- ✓ Fiber 1.1g
- ✓ Sugar 0.3g
- ✓ Protein 4.6g

Recipe 29: Keto Proof Green Tea

- o Total Time: 10 minutes
- o Serves: 1

Ingredients

- Organic green tea 2-3 teabags
- Grass-fed unsalted butter 2 tablespoons
- Coconut oil 2 tablespoons

- • Heavy cream 1 tablespoon
- • Ice cubes 3 cups

Instructions

1. Make your favorite cup of tea.

2. Add the coconut oil and butter and mix well, leaving it delicious.

3. Cool the tea in the freezer for several hours.

4. Put your ice cubes and tea into the blender.

5. Mix for 3-5 minutes, until well blended.

Nutrition

- ✓ Calories 503
- ✓ Carbs 0.43 g
- ✓ Fat 55.39 g
- ✓ Protein 0.67 g

Recipe 30: Low Carb Cucumber Green Tea Detox Smoothie

o Total Time: 5 minutes

o Serves: 2

Ingredients:

- • Water 8 ounces
- • Green tea powder 2 tsp.
- • Sliced Cucumber 1 cup
- • Ripe Avocado 2 ounces
- • Lemon juice 1 tsp.
- • Stevia liquid 1/2 cup
- • Lemon 1/2 tsp.

Instructions

1. First pour the water and green tea powder into a blender and mix it.

2. Put the remaining ingredients and mix well until smooth.

3. Sweetener to taste and change as needed.

4. Serve or refrigerate immediately when you are ready to serve.

Nutrition

- ✓ Calories 69
- ✓ Net Carbs: 3.4g
- ✓ Fat 4.6g
- ✓ Carbohydrates 6.8g
- ✓ Protein 2g

Recipe 31: Keto Cinnamon Almond Butter Shake

o   Total Time: 5 minutes

o   Serves: 1

Ingredients

- Unsweetened Nut milk, One and a half cup
- Collagen Peptides, 1 scoop
- Almond butter, 2 tbsp.
- Golden flax meal, 2 tbsp.
- Cinnamon, 1/2 tsp.
- Liquid stevia, 15 drops ·
- Almond extract, 1/8 tsp.
- Salt, 1/8 tsp.
- Ice cubes, 6–8

Instructions

Add all the components to a mixer and blend for 30 seconds or until the consistency is smooth.

Nutrition

- ✓ **Calories:** 326

✓ **Fat:** 27g

✓ **Carbohydrates:** 11g

✓ **Fiber:** 5g

✓ **Protein:** 19g

Recipe 32: Cauliflower Popcorn

o   Total Time: One and a half hour

o   Serves: 6

Ingredients

- **Cauliflower**, trimmed and cut 1
- **Egg** 1 free-range
- **Milk** 2 tbsp.
- **Parmesan** finely grated 25g
- **Garlic** granules or powder 1 tsp.
- **Thyme** leaves only 2
- **Smoked paprika** 1 tsp.
- Fresh **Bread-crumbs** 100g
- Dried **Oregano** ½ tsp.
- Salt and Freshly ground **black pepper**

Instructions

1. Prepare the cauliflower in a saucepan of salted water for two minutes or till tender.

2. Make the cauliflower golden and put it on a plate lined with tissue paper. Then you can set it to dry heat for twenty minutes.

3. Set the oven to 200C/ Gas 4.

4. Take a pot, mix the egg and milk. In another big cup, add the breadcrumbs, garlic granules, parmesan cheese, smoked paprika, thyme, and dried oregano and sprinkle well with pepper and salt.

5. Drop the cauliflower in the egg and milk mixture and blend properly, making sure that the egg is in all the cauliflower nooks and crannies. Make the cauliflower topping with the breadcrumbs and put it on the cover.

6. Organize the cauliflower on a cookie sheet in a single layer and bake in the middle of the oven for 20 minutes till it starts turning crisp and golden brown. Switch the chopped cauliflower pieces over and cook for another 10 minutes or until they are all crispy.

7. Serve while it is still warm.

Nutrition

- ✓ Calories 82.7
- ✓ Protein 4.2 g
- ✓ Carbohydrates 11.2 g
- ✓ Fat 3.6g

Recipe 33: Tropical Fruit Salad

Total Time: 10 minutes

Ingredients

- Fresh ripe **mangoes**
- pineapple chunks, fresh or canned 2 cups
- Banana, sliced 1
- **Fresh papaya**, sliced into cubes 1-2 cups
- **Kiwi fruit**, in cubes. 1-2 cups
- Fresh red seedless grapes, sliced in half 2 cups
- One **dragon fruit**, or one pear, sliced into cubes
- Optional: a handful of fresh raspberries
- Coconut milk one-fourth cup
- Freshly-squeezed lime juice 2 tbsp.

Instructions

1. Cut all the fruits except the contrasting red fruit (strawberries, raspberries, or dried cranberries) and put in a bowl.
2. Sprinkle over the lime juice and gently stir to mix. Put in the freezer for at least 30 minutes or before you decide to eat your salad.
3. Before eating, add the coconut milk and mix again. If you want spicier for your liking, sprinkle over a little more lime juice. Serve in bowls and top with some red contrasting fruit raspberries, strawberries, or dried cranberries.

Recipe 34: Santa Fe Corn Salad

o Total Time: 10 minutes

o Serves: 4

Ingredients

- Corn 3 Cans
- Red bell peppers, chopped 2
- Black beans drained and rinsed 1 Can
- Avocado, chopped 1
- Juice of 2 limes
- Extra-virgin olive oil 2 tbsp.
- Red onion, finely chopped 1/2
- Cumin 1/2 tsp.
- Green onions, sliced, for garnish   2 tbsp.

Instructions

In a big bowl, add all the ingredients together. Mix until the ingredients have been thoroughly combined and covered in a coating. Garnish with herbs and serve as needed.

Nutrition

✓ Calories 123

- ✓ Fat 1.4 g
- ✓ Carbs 28.2 g
- ✓ Protein 4.1 g

Recipe 35: Baked Potatoes

o Total Time: 30 minutes

o Serves: 2

Ingredients

- Russet Potatoes 4
- Warm water half cup
- Salt 2 tablespoon
- Vegetable oil 1 tablespoon

Instructions

1. Set the oven to 450 degrees F. Position a wire rack over an 18-inch rimmed baking dish.

2. Poke each potato six times (3 times on both sides) with a fork.

3. In a wide bowl, mix water and salt until the salt has dissolved.

4. Wrap each potato in saltwater to cover it completely, move it to a wire rack while spreading it uniformly apart.

5. Cook in a preheated oven till the center reaches 205 degrees F on an instant thermometer (potatoes will be almost soft inside when pressed).

6. Spray potatoes with vegetable oil, return to the oven and bake for 10 minutes.

7. Remove from the oven and instantly cut in the cross-section to release the steam.

8. Use the kitchen towel, twist ends and open the top as required.

Recipe 36: Crock Pot Stuffed Peppers

o Total Time: 3 hours

o Serves: 4

Ingredients

- Ground beef 1 lb.
- Black beans, drained one can
- Diced fire-roasted tomatoes, drained one can
- Shredded Monterey jack cheese, two can
- cooked white rice 1 c
- Frozen corn defrosted 1 c.
- Chili powder 1 tsp.
- Cumin 1 tsp.
- Freshly ground black pepper
- Kosher salt
- Oregano 1/2 tsp.
- Garlic powder 1/2 tsp.
- Bell peppers, tops and seeds removed 4
- Sour cream, for serving
- 1 tbsp. Chopped cilantro, for garnish.

Instructions

1. In a big bowl, mix beef with beans, onions, 1 cup of cheese, sugar, corn, cumin, chili powder, garlic powder, and oregano. Mix until all components have been thoroughly integrated. Sprinkle as per your taste with salt and pepper.

2. Stuff the beef mixture with the peppers and put them in the crock-pot, open side up. Cover and cook for 3 hours.

3. Once the peppers are soft, top them up with the remaining cheese and cover. Cook on low for 5-10 minutes or till cheese is melted.

4. Garnish and serve with cilantro and sour cream.

Nutrition

- ✓ Calories 355
- ✓ Fat 15 g
- ✓ Carbs 30 g
- ✓ Protein 27 g

Chapter 4: Lunch and Dinner Recipes for Intermittent Fasting

4.1 Delicious Recipes List that You Can Enjoy at Lunch and Dinner

Recipe 1: Avocado Quesadillas

- o Total Time:31 minutes
- o Serves: 2

Ingredients

- Vine-ripe tomatoes, seeded and chopped into 1/4-inch pieces 2

- Avocado, peeled, pitted, and chopped into 1/4-inch pieces 1 ripe

- Chopped red onion 1 tablespoon

- Fresh lemon juice 2 teaspoons

- Tabasco sauce 1/4 teaspoon

- Salt and pepper

- Sour cream 1/4 cup

- Chopped fresh coriander 3 tablespoons

- Flour tortillas 24 inches

- Vegetable oil 1/2 teaspoon

- Shredded cheese 1 1/3 cups

Instructions

1.   Mix the onions, avocado, tomato, lemon juice, and Tabasco in a small bowl.

2.   Season with salt and pepper to taste.

3.   In some other small bowl, combine the sour cream, coriander, salt, and pepper to taste.

4.   Place tortillas on a baking plate and sprinkle the tops with oil.

5.   Broil tortillas 2 to 4 inches from the flame to a golden brown.

6.   Spray tortillas generously with cheese and toast till cheese is melted.

7.   Disperse the avocado mixture smoothly over two tortillas and cover each with one of the leftover tortillas, the cheese side down to make two quesadillas.

8.   Shift the quesadillas to the cutting block and chop it into four slices.

9.   Garnish each slice with a mixture of sour cream and enjoy warm.

Nutrition

- ✓ Calories 332
- ✓ Carbs 38g
- ✓ Fat 18g
- ✓ Protein 9g
- ✓ Fiber 10g
- ✓ Net carbs 28g

Recipe 2: Cobb Salad with Brown Derby French Dressing

- o Total Time: 45 minutes
- o Serves: 6

Ingredients

- Red wine vinegar ½ cup

- Water ½ cup

- Vegetable oil ½ cup
- Olive oil ⅓ cup
- Lemon juice 1 tablespoon
- Salt 1 teaspoon
- Worcestershire sauce 1 ½ teaspoons
- Garlic, minced 1 clove
- Dry mustard ½ teaspoon
- Ground black pepper 1 teaspoon
- White sugar ½ teaspoon

For Salad

- Chopped iceberg lettuce, 1 head
- Tomatoes, chopped 3
- Watercress, trimmed and chopped, 1 bunch
- Sliced deli turkey meat, diced ¾ pound
- Cooked bacon, crumbled ½ pound
- Avocados, diced 2

Instructions

1. Mix the water, olive oil, vegetable oil, red wine vinegar, lemon juice, Worcestershire sauce, garlic, salt, pepper, sugar, and mustard in a bowl till the dressing is smooth.

2. Put the sliced lettuce and watercress in a large bowl of salad. Complete with tomatoes, turkey, eggs, blue cheese, bacon, and avocados. Until serving, add the appropriate amount of seasoning.

Nutrition

- ✓ Calories 530.4
- ✓ Protein 23.3g

✓ carbohydrates 11.6 g

✓ Fat 155.4 mg

Recipe 3: Vegan Fish Tacos

o Total Time: 20 minutes

o Serves: 4

Ingredients

• Zest and juice 2 limes

• Sea salt 1 teaspoon

• Shredded purple cabbage 3 cups

• Mango diced

• Medium red onion diced 1/2

• Soy yogurt ½ cup

• Adobo sauce 2 teaspoons

• 1 jar of hearts of palm 6 pieces

• Oil as required

• Avocado diced 1

• Baking powder 1 teaspoon

• Flour ½ cup or (64 grams)

• Ice water ½ cup

• Cilantro chopped, a small bunch

• 12 small tortillas toasted in a pan or warmed in the microwave.

Instructions

1. Place the cabbage in a bowl and pour in half a lime juice and add 1/2 teaspoon of salt. Toss to mix and refrigerate.

2. In a separate cup, mix the mango, avocado, and red onion and refrigerate them.

3. In a pan, mix the adobo sauce, soy yogurt, zest of one lime, half lime juice, and one-fourth teaspoon of salt and refrigerate them.

4. Split the hearts of the palm half lengthwise and crosswise into four parts. Give heat to the oil in a pan over medium-high heat and prepare a sheet lined with paper towels. Ensure all the taco mixes are ready, and the oil is warm before mixing.

5. In a dish, mix flour, baking powder, and one-fourth teaspoon of salt. Mix in the ice water to make a thick drum. To avoid over mixing this, it is all right if there are a few lumps in there. Put a few pieces of palm hearts and pass them to the hot oil. Cook, turning once, if needed, for a few minutes until golden brown, then transfer to a paper towel-lined plate to clean.

6. Present all the ingredients on top of the hot tortillas. You can sprinkle the sauce on top and a slathering of fresh cilantro and a wedge of lime on edge.

Nutrition

- ✓ Calories: 144
- ✓ Carbohydrates: 23g
- ✓ Protein: 3g
- ✓ Fat: 5g

Recipe 4: Mediterranean Chicken Breasts with Avocado Tapenade

o   Total Time: 15 minutes

o   Serves: 4

Ingredients

- Lemon peel Grated 1

- Garlic clove 1

- Salt, to taste

- Lemon juice 5 tbsp.

- Skinless and Boneless chicken 4 halves

- Pepper one-fourth tsp.

- Olive oil 2 tbsp.

- Tomato 1 medium

- Sea salt half teaspoon

- Capers 3tbsp.

- Green Pimento stuffed olive, one-fourth cup

- Basil leaves 2tbsp.

Instructions

1. In a sealed plastic bag, mix chicken and lemon peel, marinade, two tablespoons of olive oil, two tablespoons of lemon juice, garlic, salt, and pepper. Seal and refrigerate the bag for 30 minutes.

2. In a container, mix the left-over three tablespoons of lemon juice, roasted garlic, remaining half teaspoons of olive oil, sea salt, and fresh ground pepper. Mix in tomatoes, capers, green olives, basil, and avocado; set aside.

3. Take the chicken from the bag and remove the marinade. Roast over medium-hot coals for 4 to 5 minutes per side or at the desired degree of crispiness.

4. Serve with the Tapenade of Avocado.

Nutrition

- ✓ Calories277
- ✓ Fat 16.4g
- ✓ Carbs 6.9g
- ✓ Protein 26g

Recipe 5: Sauerkraut Salad

- o Total Time: 15 minutes along with cooling time
- o Serves: 10 to 12

Ingredients

- Grated carrots 1 cup
- Diced pimientos, drained one jar
- Sauerkraut washed one can
- Chopped green pepper 1 cup
- Chopped onion 1 cup
- Chopped celery 1 cup
- Canola oil 1/2 cup
- Sugar 3/4 cup

Instructions

Combine the sauerkraut, celery, carrots, onion, green pepper, and paprika in a large bowl. In a medium bowl or jar, combine sugar and oil. Put over the vegetables and combine well. Cover and put in the freezer for at least eight hours.

Nutrition

- ✓ Calories 19
- ✓ Fat 0.1 g
- ✓ Carbs 4.7 g
- ✓ Protein 0.9 g

Recipe 6: Tilapia Parmesan

- o Total Time: 17 minutes
- o Serves: 4

Ingredients

- Lemon juice 2 tablespoons
- Grated parmesan cheese 1/2 cup

- Tilapia fillets 4
- Butter, room temperature 2 tablespoons
- Mayonnaise 3 tablespoons
- Seasoning salt one-fourth teaspoon
- Dried basil one-fourth teaspoon
- Finely chopped green onions 3 tablespoons
- Black pepper
- Hot pepper sauce 1 dash

Instructions

1. Set the oven to 350 degrees.

2. Put the filets in a single layer in a buttered thirteen by nine-inch baking dish or jelly roll pan. Brush the surface with some juice.

3. In a bowl, add cheese, butter, mayonnaise, onion, and seasonings. Mix well.

4. Bake the fish for 5 minutes on each side or until it is almost done, depending on the size.

5. Top with the cheese mixture and fry another 2 to 3 minutes or till browned.

Nutrition

- ✓ Calories 202
- ✓ Fat 11.5 g
- ✓ Carbs 0.2 g
- ✓ Protein 23.7g

Recipe 7: Street Tacos

o   Total Time: 5

o   Serves:1

Ingredients

- Black beans, heated up 1/4 cup

- Red onion, diced 1/2 cup

- Cooked grass-fed beef 4 oz.

- Salsa one-fourth cup

- Red bell pepper, diced 1

- Cilantro, diced 1/4 cup

- Romaine lettuce leaves 4 or corn tortillas

- Guacamole 1/4 cup

Instructions

Make the topping of all the items on the corn tortillas or the romaine lettuce.

Nutrition

- ✓ Calories 100
- ✓ Fat 4 g
- ✓ Carbs 9 g
- ✓ Protein 10 g

Recipe 8: Roasted Cauliflower Tahini

- o Total Time: 1 hour
- o Serves: 4-6

Ingredients

- Cauliflower Florets 2 lbs.

- Tahini 2 tbsp.

- Avocado Oil 2 tbsp.

- Sea Salt, to taste

- Lemon Juice 2 tsp.

Instructions

1. Settle the oven to 400 degrees F in a heat transfer bake environment. Sprinkle the cauliflower flowers with one tablespoon of avocado oil on a large baking tray lined with parchment paper. Sauté till mixed.

2. Bake till the cauliflower becomes brown and crisp, approximately 20 minutes, stir once to confirm even browning.

3. When the cauliflower gets roasted, mix the lemon juice, tahini, and the leftover avocado oil.

4. Cover the roasted cauliflower in the lemon tahini sauce. Transfer the cauliflower to the oven and cook the tahini sauce for about 5 minutes.

5. Sprinkle roasted cauliflower with sea salt as your taste needs. Serve right away.

Nutrition

- ✓ Calories 79
- ✓ Carbs 6g
- ✓ Fat 6g
- ✓ Protein 3g

Recipe 9: Roasted Vegetable Soup

- o Total Time: 1 hour and 30 minutes
- o Serves: 3-4

Ingredients

- Zucchini, in three-fourth inch pieces 2 medium
- Eggplant, in three-fourth inch pieces 1 medium
- Fresh mushrooms, 1/2 pound
- Sweet red peppers, cut in three-fourth inch pieces 2 large

- potato, peeled and cut into three-fourth inch pieces 1 large

- Vegetable or chicken broth 4 cans

- Garlic cloves, minced 2

- Kidney beans, rinsed and drained 1 can

- Sweet potato, peeled in three-fourth inch pieces 1 large

- Black-eyed peas, rinsed 1 can

- Leek (only white part), sliced 1 medium

- Garbanzo beans or chickpeas, rinsed and drained 1 can

- Red wine vinegar 2 to 3 teaspoons

- Dried rosemary, crushed 1 teaspoon

- Dried marjoram 1 teaspoon

- Rubbed sage 1/2 teaspoon

- Dried thyme 1/2 teaspoon

- Pepper and salt to taste

Instructions

1. Put the foil in two baking pans.

2. Cover the foil with cooking grease.

3. Put zucchini, eggplant, leek, peppers, potatoes, and mushrooms on pans. Then spray well to coat. Bake, without covering, on 425° for about twenty-five to thirty minutes or till tender.

4.   With the help of a cooking spray coat in a Dutch oven, cook garlic for around 2 minutes. Then put broth, peas, beans, vinegar, roasted vegetables and seasonings. Wait for it to boil. Decrease the flame heat; put a cover and mix for around 10 to12 minutes or till cooked.

Nutrition

- ✓ Calories 149.9
- ✓ Fat 2.8 g
- ✓ Carbs 23 g
- ✓ Protein 9.2 g

Recipe 10: Cauliflower Tabbouleh and Falafel Chicken Patties

- o Total Time: 12 minutes
- o Serves: 4

Ingredients

- Flat leaf parsley 1 cup
- Florets of Cauliflower 3 cups
- Cucumber diced 1
- Lemon juice 2 tablespoon
- Tomato 1
- Green onions 3
- Olive oil 1 tablespoon
- Pepper one-fourth tsp.
- Salt half teaspoon

Falafel Chicken Patties

- Garlic clove, 1
- Ground chicken 450 g
- Parsley, cut 1 tbsp.
- Chickpea flour 2 tbsp.
- Onion powder 1 tsp.
- Cumin half tsp.
- Vegetable oil 2 tbsp.

- Salt one-fourth tsp.

Instructions

Cauliflower Tabbouleh

1. Flutter florets of cauliflower in a food blender until they are the size of rice grains.

2. Then take a large utensil, whisk cauliflower rice, cucumber, parsley, green onion, and tomato.

3. Mix, oil, lemon juice, pepper, and salt in a small bowl. Mix in the mixture of cauliflower.

Falafel Chicken Patties

1. Whisk ground chicken with chickpea flour, garlic, parsley, cumin salt, and onion powder in a bowl. Properly separate the mixture into four and transform into three-fourth inch thickness patties.

2. Warm the oil in a utensil over moderate to high flame. Toast patties in the pan till golden and cooked properly, about five to six minutes each side.

3. Serve cauliflower Tabbouleh along with falafel chicken patties.

Nutrition

- ✓ Calories 68
- ✓ Fat 3.8 g
- ✓ Protein 2.6 g

Recipe 11: Spanish Meatballs in Chipotle Sauce

- o Total Time: 30 minutes
- o Serves: 4

Ingredients

Meatballs:

- Ground meat 500 g
- Garlic cloves 2
- 1 egg
- Dried breadcrumbs 2 ½ tablespoons
- Parsley cut 2 tablespoons
- Sweet paprika three-fourth teaspoon
- Hot paprika one-fourth teaspoon
- Salt 1 teaspoon
- Smoked paprika one-fourth teaspoon
- Black pepper one-fourth teaspoon
- Olive oil 1 tablespoon

Tomato sauce:

- Olive oil 2 tablespoons
- Garlic cloves 3
- Medium onion 1
- 2 cans chopped tomatoes
- ½ teaspoon fennel seeds
- Cayenne pepper one-fourth teaspoon
- Dried oregano1 teaspoon
- 2 bay leaves
- Pepper and salt

Instructions

Meatballs:

1. Put the minced meat, ground cloves of garlic, dried breadcrumbs, parsley, slightly beaten egg, sweet, smoked and pepper, salt, hot paprika in a pot. Whisk enough with the hand manually. Make around 30 to 35 smaller size meatballs around the walnut size.

2. Warm the oil in a large pot. Fry the meatballs (in two segments) till brownish evenly on the sides. It will need almost 5 minutes. Remove the meatballs from the pot and put them separately.

Tomato Sauce:

1. Cut the onion very smoothly.

2. Warm two tablespoons of olive oil in that pan you used earlier. Put the onion and cook it until golden. Put the smoothly cut garlic cloves and whisk for one more minute.

3. Put the tomatoes from the tin, bay leaves, oregano, cayenne pepper, chopped parsley, and fennel seeds. Put some pepper and salt as well. Mix well and bring it to a boil. Simmer on medium-low heat for 20 minutes or until slightly thickened.

4. Add the meatballs to the pan and warm them in the sauce for around 5 minutes or till cooked properly and present it.

Nutrition

- ✓ Calories 565
- ✓ Fat 38 g
- ✓ Carbs 12 g
- ✓ Protein 43 g

Recipe 12: Broccoli Detox Soup

- o Total Time: 25 minutes
- o Serves: 4

Ingredients

- Celery stalks finely diced 2 cups

- Broccoli florets 2 cups

- Garlic cloves crushed 2

- Onion chopped 1

- Parsnip peeled 1

- Filtered water 2 cups
- Carrot peeled and finely chopped 1
- Greens kale, spinach, or beet greens 1 cup
- Sea salt half tsp
- Coconut oil 1 tsp.
- Lemon juice half
- Mixed seeds and nuts 1 teaspoon
- Chia seeds 1 tbsp.
- Coconut milk, for garnishing

Instructions

1. Take a pot for soup, warm the coconut oil, add garlic, onion, carrot, celery sticks, broccoli, and parsnip, and cook on low flame heat for about 5 minutes, mixing regularly.

2. Put the water or broth of vegetable, wait till a boil, then put a cover on the pot and let cook for five to seven minutes, till the vegetables are juicy but not smashed.

3. Mix in the green veggies, then shift into the processor, put the lemon, and chia seeds, and process to get a fine cream.

4. Put toasted seeds on the top and serve warm.

Nutrition

- ✓ Calories 182
- ✓ Fat 4.2g
- ✓ Carbs 35g
- ✓ Protein 5.5g

Recipe 13: Berry Crisp

O Total Time: 15 minutes

o Serves: 1

Ingredients

- Fresh blackberries one-fourth cup
- fresh raspberries one-fourth cup
- Light brown sugar 2 teaspoons
- Ground cinnamon one pinch
- Low-fat granola cereal 2 tablespoons

Instructions

1. Settle the oven to 400 degrees F and sprinkle through cooking spray an eight oz.in ramekin

2. Put the brown sugar, berries, and cinnamon to the ramekin and whisk to mix.

3. Spray the granola cereal on the berry mixture.

4. Toast for around 10 minutes.

5. Present warm.

Nutrition

- ✓ Calories 154
- ✓ Carbs 28 g
- ✓ Protein 3 g
- ✓ Fat 3 g

Recipe 14: Roasted Veggies Farro Salad

o   Total Time: 40 minutes

o   Serves: one to two as a main dish

Ingredients

- Cooked farro 1½ cups
- Broccoli florets ⅔ cup
- Grape tomatoes, halved one-fourth cup
- Zucchini, cut one-fourth
- Bell pepper, chopped half
- Olive oil 1 tsp

- Sea salt 1 tsp
- Dried or fresh rosemary 1 tsp
- Garlic, minced 1 clove
- kalamata olives, sliced 4-5
- Walnut halves, chopped one-fourth cup
- Crumbled goat cheese 2 tbsp.

Instructions

1. Settle the oven to 400°F and layer parchment paper on the pan.

2. Cook, tomatoes, broccoli, bell pepper, and zucchini with olive oil, rosemary, salt and minced garlic in a pot till finely covered.

3. Scatter in the ready pan and cook in the settled oven for around 25 minutes.

4. Mix warmed vegetables with toasted farro, diced olives, and walnuts.

5. Put salt as your taste.

6. For topping, use crumbled goat cheese.

Nutrition

- ✓ Calories: 315 kcals
- ✓ Fat 13 g
- ✓ Carbohydrates: 37.5 g
- ✓ Fiber: 7.5 g
- ✓ Protein 8 g

Recipe 15: Cajun Potato, Avocado, and Shrimp/ Prawn Salad

o   Total Time: 30mins

o   Serves: 2

Ingredients

- New Potatoes 300g
- Olive oil 1 tbsp.
- King prawns 250 g
- Garlic clove 1
- Cajun seasoning 2 tsp.
- Alfalfa 1
- Onion springs 2
- Avocado 1
- Salt a little bit for boiling potatoes

Instructions

1. Toast the potatoes in a big pot of slightly salted boiling water for ten to fifteen minutes or until tender, drain well.

2. Warm the oil in a pot or nonstick frying pan.

3. Add the prawns, garlic, spring onions and Cajun seasoning and stir fry for two to three minutes or until the prawns are hot.

4. Stir in the potatoes and cook for a further minute.

5. Transfer to serving dishes and top with avocado and alfalfa sprouts and serve.

Nutrition Information

- ✓ Calories 435
- ✓ Carbs 37.9g
- ✓ Fat 23g
- ✓ Protein 23.1g

Recipe 16: Baked Mahi (Fish)

Total Time: 30 minutes

Serves: 2

Ingredients

- Fillets of fish 4
- Salt one-eight tsp.
- Unsalted butter 3 tbsp.
- Pepper one-eight tsp.
- Minced garlic 1/4 tsp.
- Lemon juice 3 tsp.
- Lemon 1

Instructions

1. Settle the oven to 425 degrees F.

2. Line a baking sheet with parchment, then oil the paper with cooking spray or sprinkle the olive oil.

3. Put the defrost fillets of fish over the parchment sheet. Sprinkle it with pepper and salt.

4. Warm the butter, then put the minced garlic along with lemon juice and mix to combine.

5. By the help of a bashing brush, put the lemon butter mixture on the fillets of Mahi.

6. Cut one lemon into thin pieces, extract any seeds and place onto the fillets.

7. Cook for about 20 minutes or till the fillets are flaky and reach an internal temperature of 137 degrees F.

8. Remove from the oven. Using the basting brush, brush the melted lemon butter from the pan over the fillets once again. Serve it.

Nutrition

- ✓ Calories 104
- ✓ Total Fat 8.9g
- ✓ Total Carbohydrate 1g
- ✓ Protein 5.4g

Recipe 17: Broccoli Dal Curry

- o Total Time: 20 minutes
- o Serves: 3

Ingredients

- Broccoli 8-10 florets
- Curd 2 tablespoon
- Fresh cream 2 tablespoon
- Turmeric powder 1 teaspoon
- Coriander powder 1 teaspoon
- Black pepper half teaspoon
- Cumin seeds powder half teaspoon
- Red chili in powdered form half teaspoon
- Garlic cloves 4
- Green Chili 2
- Salt as your taste
- Olive Oil 1 tablespoon
- Ginger half inch piece
- Tomato roughly chopped 1
- Onion 1 finely chopped

Instructions

1. Have some water in a wide utensil and wait to boil on high heat.

2. Put florets of broccoli to it and wait for it to boil in water for some time unless they soften.

3. After that switch off the flame and remove the broccoli florets from the hot water.

4. Shift these florets to a utensil of cold water. It helps the broccoli to maintain its fresh color and gets soft and juicy.

5. Take a big pot, put tomato, green chilies, ginger, and garlic cloves.

6. Mix all the components making a smooth paste.

7. Shift the prepared mixture to a bowl and put the spices and salt as per taste to it.

8. Combine all the components to form a uniform spice paste for the gravy.

9. Warm a tablespoon of olive oil in a pot.

10. Put chopped onion into it. Toast the chopped onions until they turn golden in shade.

11. Put the spice mixture into this pot and mix well to cook the spices.

12. As the oil starts to scatter from the spices then put curd to the pot.

13. Mix frequently to prevent any block formation.

14. After that, put fresh cream and whisk to combine all the components well to make a smooth creamy curry.

15. Now put a big cup of water in the curry.

16. As the curry starts to boil, decrease the heat to medium flame and cook for five minutes. Then switch off the heat.

17. Fresh and delicious broccoli curry is ready to present.

Nutrition

- ✓ Calories 444
- ✓ Total Fat 15.4 g
- ✓ Total Carbohydrate 59 g
- ✓ Protein 25.7 g

Recipe 18: Chicken and Brussel Sprout

- o   Total Time: 40mins
- o   Serves: 4

Ingredients

- Oregano 2 tbsp.
- Garlic cloves 2
- Red onion 1
- Extra virgin olive oil 4 tbsp.
- Ground pepper half tsp.
- Brussel sprouts 1 pound
- Gnocchi package 1
- Boneless chicken thighs 4
- Red-wine vinegar 1 tbsp.
- Cherry Tomatoes 1 cup

Instructions

1. Settle the oven at 450 F.

2. In a big bowl, mix two tablespoons of oil, one tablespoon of oregano, half of the garlic, 1/4 teaspoon of pepper, and 1/8 teaspoon of salt. Add the Brussels sprouts, gnocchi, and onion, twist to cover. Set over a baking sheet.

3. Mix 1 tablespoon of butter, the leftover garlic, one tablespoon of oregano, and the leftover one-fourth teaspoon of pepper and one-fourth teaspoon of salt in a wide pot.

4. Put the chicken and cover it with a lid.

5. Place the chicken in the vegetable mixture.

6. Cook for about ten minutes.

7. Take from the oven and put tomatoes, whisk to mix.

8. Continue to cook till the Brussels sprouts are tender, and the chicken is cooked through, in about 10 minutes longer.

9. Stir the vinegar and the remaining one tablespoon of oil into the vegetable mixture.

Nutrition

- ✓ Calories 351
- ✓ Fat 15.4 g
- ✓ Carbs 24.7 g
- ✓ Protein 28.6 g

Recipe 19: Cauliflower Pizza Crust

o   Total Time: 1 hour

o   Serves: six to eight

Ingredients

- Florets of Cauliflower 2 pound
- Beaten egg 1
- Mozzarella cheese half cup
- Dried oregano
- Himalayan salt one-fourth tsp.

Instructions

1. Settle the oven to 400 degrees F.

2. Pulse batches of raw cauliflower flowers in a food processor till a rice-like consistency is achieved. Yet do not over-cream or process it.

3. Microwave the cauliflower rice for around 1 minute till it is tender. Boil it in a big pot, load it with about an inch of water, and bring it to a simmer.

4. Put the rice cauliflower and cover. Process for 4-5 minutes.

5. When the cauliflower is cooked, pour into a fine strainer or over a cloth of cheese.

6. Place a fine-mesh cheesecloth on your towel counter. Add the mixture to the cloth of the cheese and use the cheesecloth. Catch and expel any excess moisture into the drain. Take out more moisture by patting the towel again. Ensure all the water gets removed by pulling the cloth out.

7. Once the moisture has been separated, pass the "rice" to a large mixing bowl.

8. Put the beaten eggs, oregano, cheese, and salt. You can do hand blending.

9. Press the dough onto a baking sheet lined with parchment paper. Place the hands flat and place the sides to form a one-third inch high shape. Get a little higher on the hands.

10. Continue the baking regime for 35-40 minutes at 400 degrees F or till the crust is firm and golden brown.

11. After removing from the oven, make a topping. Bake for five to ten more minutes till the cheese is soft and slimy. Serve right away.

Nutrition

- ✓ Calories 56
- ✓ Fat 2.6 g
- ✓ Carbs 4.1 g
- ✓ Protein 4.8 g

Recipe 20: Black Beans and Sweet Potato Burritos

O Total Time: 55 minutes

O Serves: 6

Ingredients

- Jalapeno, seeded and finely diced 1
- Sweet potatoes, peeled and cubed small 2
- Small red onion, diced small 1
- Olive oil 2 teaspoons

- Chili powder 1 teaspoon
- Red pepper, diced small 1
- Cumin 1 teaspoon
- Salt half teaspoon
- Black pepper one-fourth teaspoon
- Can of black beans, rinsed and drain
- Fresh lime juice (from about 1 lime) 2 teaspoons
- Shredded Monterey Jack cheese 1 cup
- Burrito-size tortillas 6-8
- Shredded cheddar cheese 1 cup
- Chopped cilantro one-fourth to half cup
- Can of black beans, rinsed and drain 1

Instructions

1. Set the oven to 425F temperature.

2. In a big bowl, mix the sweet potatoes, jalapeno, red pepper, and red onion with the olive oil, cumin, chili powder, salt, and pepper.

3. Put the seasoned vegetables onto a large baking tray and cook for 18-20 minutes, flipping halfway through.

4. When the cooking process ends, the veggies should be soft but not smashed.

5. Let the mixture of vegetables cool. Split the mixture into a broad bowl and add black beans, cilantro, and lime juice. Flavor the mixture and include salt and pepper to taste, if necessary. Please put it in the fridge until the burritos are available instantly

6. Put 3-4 tortillas on a microwave-safe dish and cover with a damp paper towel. Microwave for 15-20 seconds until the tortillas are foldable. Layer one-fourth cup of the vegetable mixture in the center of the tortilla.

7. Then make a topping with a sprinkle of shredded cheese, a little of each kind. Fold in the sides of the tortilla and roll it up. Place your seam-side down on a baking sheet. Repeat the remaining tortillas until you have all the burritos you need (you can put the filling in the refrigerator and use it for 3-4 days).

8. Keep in a 375 F temperature set oven for around 10-15 minutes to bake till the top of the tortilla is golden brown. Adjust the baking time as appropriate, depending on whether or not the filling has been refrigerated. For a softer tortilla, cover each burrito in tin foil and heat it. Serve right away.

Nutrition

- ✓ Calories 542
- ✓ Fat 12g
- ✓ Carbs 95g
- ✓ Fiber 17g
- ✓ Sugar 15g
- ✓ Protein 16g

Recipe 21: Black-Eyed Peas Over a Slow Cooker

o   Total Time: 10 hours

o   Serves: 6

Ingredients

- Chicken bouillon cubes 2
- Dried black-eyed peas 1
- Water 6 cups
- Yellow onion quartered half
- Smoked ham hock 1
- Garlic Cloves smashed 2
- Salt 1 teaspoon

Instructions

1. Pick and wash the peas, remove any discolored peas.

2. Add peas, water, salt, onion, ham, buckwheat cubes, and garlic, and a slow cooker of 4 to 6-quarter. Cook on a low flame for around eight to ten hours or at a high flame for five to six hours.

Nutrition

- ✓ Calories 304
- ✓ Fat 24g
- ✓ Carbs 8g
- ✓ Protein 12g

Recipe 22: Sweet Potato, Chickpea and Spinach Curry

- o Total Time: 50 minutes
- o Serves: 5

Ingredients

- Brown onion peeled and finely chopped 1
- Olive or coconut oil 1 Tbsp.
- Tomato puree 2 Tbsp.
- Garlic cloves peeled and crushed 2
- Curry powder 1 Tbsp.
- Ground cumin 1 1/2 tsp
- Hot spices 2 tsp
- Coriander 2 tsp
- Fresh ginger peeled and grated a piece of 2- inch
- Large sweet potatoes peeled and diced 2
- Dried fenugreek leaves optional 2 Tbsp.
- Creamed coconut 100 g
- Tin chopped tomatoes 400 g
- Water 300 - 600 ml

- Tins chickpeas drained 2 400 g
- Salt to taste
- Frozen spinach 350 g
- Fresh coriander finely chopped a handful

Instructions

1. Warm the oil in a broad pan, add chopped onion and fry to low heat for about 10 minutes until soft.

2. Put ginger, garlic, curry powder, cumin, tomato purée, coriander, and hot spices and Sauté for a few more minutes.

3. Put tinned tomatoes, creamed coconut, fenugreek leaves, and 300ml water and bring to a boil.

4. Whisk unless the creamed coconut gets melted.

5. Put the sweet potato and cook for 15 minutes, unless it gets tender. Put more water as needed.

6. Add chickpeas and spinach.

7. Simmer for another 10 minutes till the sweet potatoes are tender.

8. Mix in the chopped cilantro and season them generously with salt. Serve with some pasta.

Nutrition

- ✓ Calories: 166.5
- ✓ Total Fat 2.4 g
- ✓ Total Carbohydrate 32 g
- ✓ Protein 6.8 g

Recipe 23: Millet and Quinoa Mediterranean Salad

- o Total Time: 40 minutes
- o Serves: 4

Ingredients

- Water **one and a half cup**
- Millet **1/2 cup**
- Quinoa (red, white, or black) **1/2 cup**
- Water **3/4 cup**
- Cucumber, diced 1
- Sweet pepper, seeded, diced 1
- **Red** onion, sliced **thin 1/2**
- Garlic clove, pressed **2**
- Tomato, ripe **,** seeds squeezed out, diced 1
- Cayenne pepper (more **, to taste) 1/4 tsp**
- Pine nuts **one-fourth cup**
- Feta cheese, crushed 200g
- **Can of large** white beans, drained 1
- Dried dill **(** sub basil **or** oregano, if preferred) **2 tsp**
  Lemon **,** juice **1**
- Olive oil **(optional) 1 tbsp.**
- Fresh ground pepper **, to taste**

Instructions

1. Take millet and a cup of water and make a boil.

2. Decrease heat and simmer for 5 minutes. Then turn off the flame, put a cover, and let it stay for 10 minutes.

3. Let quinoa and a three-fourth cup of water boil, decrease heat and cook, and cover 12-14 minutes till fluffy.

4. Combine all ingredients by flipping.

5. Cool it and savor it!

Nutrition

- ✓ Calorie 641
- ✓ Fat 25.7 g
- ✓ Carbs 78 g
- ✓ Protein27 g

Recipe 24: Garlic Baked Brie

- o Total Time: 20 minutes
- o Serves: 4

Ingredients

- Brie 200g
- Sage Leaves or your herb of choice 4 to 6
- Garlic Cloves, chopped 3 to 4
-

Instructions

1. Set the oven to a temperature of 180C.

2. Place the brie on the ovenproof plate.

3. Grade the top of the brie and fill the gaps with the diced garlic.

4. Cover with the leaves of the sage.

5. Put in the already settled oven for 15 to 20 minutes or till cooked to your taste.

6. Present as it is or as part of a cheese platter or cucumber, with celery, or cocktail sausages for dipping.

Nutrition

- ✓ Calories 118
- ✓ Carbs 4g
- ✓ Protein 6g
- ✓ Fat 9g

Recipe 25: Pumpkin Carrot Soup

O Total Time: 45 minutes

O Serves: 6

Ingredients

- Olive oil, 1 tbsp.
- sugar pumpkin, 2 3/4 lb.
- carrot 1 lb.
- onion, thinly sliced 1
- Fresh sage sprigs 2
- cloves garlic, thinly sliced 2
- Pepper and Kosher salt
- Nutmeg Pinch

Instructions

1. Warm 1 tablespoon of oil in a big pot over medium heat. Add the pumpkin, onion, carrots, sage, garlic, and a half tsp. of each salt and pepper and cook, covered, stirring off and on until tender for 12 minutes. Stir in the nutmeg; cook for 1 minute.

2. Put five cups of water and wait for a boil, then simmer for five to seven minutes until vegetables are tender. Drop the sage and use an immersion blender (or a regular blender, in chunks), purée the broth until pure.

3. In the meantime, heat the oven to 400 ° F. Place the reserved pumpkin seeds with the remaining 2 tsp. of oil on a rimmed baking sheet and a pinch of each salt and pepper and cook, stirring once, until golden brown and crisp for 18 to 20 minutes. Serve the soup topped with seeds and if desired, drizzle with olive oil.

Nutrition

- ✓ Calories 240

Recipe 26: Cajun Red Beans and Rice

- o Total Time: 30 minutes
- o Serves: 5

Ingredients

- Olive oil 3 tablespoons
- Garlic, minced 3 cloves
- Salt ½ teaspoon
- Large onion, chopped 1
- Chopped green bell pepper ½ cup
- Celery, including green leaves, chopped 1 stalk
- Cumin 1 teaspoon
- Thyme ½ teaspoon
- Cooked rice 20½ cups
- Chili powder 1 tablespoon
- 15-ounce cans dark red kidney beans, 2
- Fresh parsley for garnish

Instructions

1. In a large utensil, warm the olive oil. Make the preparation of garlic, bell pepper, onions, and celery in oil over medium heat until the onions are golden (almost 7 minutes). Include salt, chili cumin, and thyme.

2. Add beans and stir well. Decrease the heat to a minimum flame and keep cooking for some more minutes till the beans are dry. You must whisk regularly to avoid stuffing.

3. Put the rice into the bean mixture and blend well with all the ingredients. Cook the rice for five minutes before serving. Marinate with sprigs of parsley, enjoy.

Nutrition

- ✓ Calories 336
- ✓ Fat 8.4g
- ✓ Carbs 51g
- ✓ Protein 12g

Recipe 27: Grilled Lemon Salmon

O Total Time: 50 minutes

O Serves: 4

Ingredients

- Fresh dill 2teaspoons
- Pepper ½ teaspoon
- Salt ½ teaspoon
- Garlic powder ½ teaspoon
- Salmon fillets 1 ½ lbs.
- Chicken bouillon cube, 1
- Water 3 tablespoons
- Soy sauce 3 tablespoons
- Packed brown sugar ¼ cup
- Thinly sliced lemon, 1
- Oil 3 tablespoons
- Finely chopped green onions 4 tablespoons
- Thinly sliced lemon, 1
- Onions, separated into rings 2 slices

Instructions

1. Slather with the dill, salt, pepper, and garlic powder over the salmon.

2. Put it in a wide glass container.

3. Combine sugar, chicken bouillon, soya sauce, milk and green onions.

4. Put the salmon.

5.   Coat and cool for 1 hour, shift once.

6.   Remove the marinade and discard it.

7.   Place on the medium heat on the grill, put the lemon and the onion on top.

8.   Put a cover and cook for 15 minutes or unless the fish is finished.

Nutrition

- ✓ Calories 386.2
- ✓ Total Fat 18.9g
- ✓ Protein 46.1g
- ✓ Carbohydrates 5.3g

Recipe 28: Crispy Brussels Sprouts with Pistachio Sage

- o Total Time: 35 minutes
- o Serves: 4

Ingredients

- Pistachios, shelled 1/4 cup
- Brussels Sprouts, cleaned and cut in half, 1 lb.
- Fresh Sage, finely chopped 2 tbsp.
- Sea Salt, to taste
- Avocado Oil 2 tbsp.

Instructions

1. Set the oven to 400 degrees F on the heat transfer bake setting. Then over a large baking tray, sprinkle brussels sprouts with one tablespoon of avocado oil. Lightly mix till combined.

2. Cook unless the Brussels sprouts get brown and crunchy on the outer side and juicy from the inner side, approximately 25 minutes, tossing the pan repeatedly to confirm uniform browning.

3. When the Brussels sprouts are cooked, smoothly cut the pistachios by utilizing a food processor or a knife, and cut the fresh leaves of sage.

4. Warm the leftover avocado oil on the moderate heating flame in a hard-frying pan like cast iron. Put nicely cut sage to warmed oil and fry for about one minute. Put pistachios into the mixture of sage oil and cook till golden brownish in look, approximately one to two minutes. Take off sauce mixture from the flame.

5. Once Brussels sprouts get completely roasted, put the pan back on moderate to high flame for warming the sage sauce of pistachio. Then put cooked Brussels sprouts and mix slowly to cover in the pistachio mixture of sage finely. Serve it now.

Nutrition

- ✓ Calories 147
- ✓ Fat 11g
- ✓ Carbs 10g
- ✓ Protein 5g

Recipe 29: Cajun Chicken Alfredo

- o Total Time: 25 minutes
- o Serves: 6

Ingredients:

- Olive oil, divided 2 tbsp.
- Green peppers, chopped 2
- Water 2 cups
- Heavy whipping cream 2 cups
- Shredded Parmesan cheese 1 cup
- Boneless chicken breasts (6 oz. each), cubed 2
- Cajun seasoning, divided 2 tbsp.
- Bow tie pasta 16 oz.
- Chicken stock 3 cups

Instructions

1. Sauté peppers in oil for 3-4 minutes and then remove them.

2. Sauté chicken and half Cajun seasoning for 3-4 minutes.

3. Add pasta, stock, and water.

4. Pressure Cook on High for 6 minutes then remove.

5. Sauté cream, Parmesan cheese, remaining Cajun seasoning, and cooked peppers.

6. Serve chicken with sauce and pasta.

Nutrition

- ✓ Calories 1250
- ✓ Carbs 129g
- ✓ Fat 86g
- ✓ Protein 66g

Recipe 30: Garlic butter Brazilian Steak

- o Total Time: 15 minutes
- o Serves: 4

Ingredients:

- Garlic 6 medium cloves

- kosher salt

- Skirt steak, trimmed into four pieces 1.5 lb.

- Freshly ground black pepper

- Canola oil or vegetable oil two tablespoons

- Unsalted butter (4 tablespoons) 2 oz.

- Chopped fresh flat-leaf parsley One tablespoon

Instructions

1. Take off the outer covering and grind the garlic cloves with the side of a knife. Sprinkle with salt and chop the garlic into thin slices.

2. Make the steak dry and sprinkle with salt and pepper evenly on both sides.

3. Warm the oil over medium-high heat in a 12-inch heavy-duty skillet until it shines hot.

4. Put the steak and make it brown well on both sides, for about 2 to 3 minutes per side.

5. Shift the steak to a plate and let the garlic butter rest before cooking it.

6. Warm the butter at low heat in an 8-inch pan.

7. Put the garlic and simmer till lightly golden, shaking the pan frequently for about 4 minutes. Add salt according to taste.

8. Slice the steak and move to four plates if you like. Spoon the steak with the garlic butter, scatter with the parsley and eat.

Nutrition

- ✓ Calories 429
- ✓ Fat 31g
- ✓ Carbohydrates 2g

Recipe 31: Chicken Enchilada Bowl

- o Total Time: 50 minutes
- o Serves: 4

Ingredients:

- Coconut oil (for searing chicken) 2 tablespoons

- Boneless, skinless chicken thighs 1 pound

- Red enchilada sauce 3/4 cup

- Water 1/4 cup

- Chopped onion one-fourth cup

- Diced green chilies 1– 4 oz.

- Avocado, diced 1
- Shredded cheese 1 cup
- Chopped pickled jalapenos 1/4 cup
- Sour cream 1/2 cup
- One tomato, chopped

Instructions

1. Warm the coconut oil in a pan or Dutch oven over moderate heat.

2. Cook thighs of chicken till lightly brown and dry.

3. Pour in the sauce and water of the enchilada and add the onion and green chilies.

4. Reduce heat and cover to low heat.

5. Toast chicken for 17-25 minutes till chicken is tender and completely cooked, do it on an internal temperature of 165 degrees.

6. Take of the chicken carefully and put it on a working surface. Chop or shred (your preference) meat, then add it back to the bowl. Let the chicken simmer and uncover to absorb flavor for another 10 minutes and allow the sauce to shrink a little.

7. Before eating, top with tomatoes, avocado, jalapeno, milk, sour cream, and any other toppings you choose. Easy to tailor to your taste. If required, just be sure to update your personal nutrition information if appropriate; serve alone or over cauliflower rice.

Nutrition

- ✓ Calories: 568kcal
- ✓ Carbohydrates: 6.14g
- ✓ Protein: 38.38g

Recipe 32: Mexican Tempeh

- o Total Time: 45 minutes
- o Serves: 6

Ingredients

- Tempeh, crumbled 8 oz.
- Olive oil 3 tablespoons
- Cumin 1 teaspoon
- Yellow onion, chopped half
- Green bell pepper, chopped 1
- Dried oregano 1 teaspoon
- Chopped cremini mushrooms half cup
- Small zucchini, chopped 1
- Cloves of garlic, minced 2
- Salsa 1/3 cup
- Chopped green chilies 1can
- Vegetable broth 3/4 cup
- Diced fire-roasted tomatoes 1
- Uncooked quinoa, rinsed 1/2 cup
- Black beans, drained and rinsed 1 can
- Frozen corn 2/3 cup
- Salt and ground black pepper, to taste
- Shredded cheddar cheese 1 cup
- Chopped cilantro for garnish

Instructions

1. Place two tbsp. olive oil in a pot for heating it.

2. Put crumbled tempeh, oregano, and cumin.

3. Mix and toast till tempeh becomes slightly browned for around 5-7 minutes.

4. Shift to the bowl and set aside.

5. Put another one tbs. of olive oil in the same pot. Put the cabbage, mushrooms, green bell pepper, and zucchini.

6. Toast for about 3-5 minutes or till the onion is translucent.

7. Mix in the onions, garlic, salsa, broth, green peppers, and the quinoa.

8. Wait for its boil and put a cover on it. Cook for about 15 minutes, stirring periodically.

9. Take off the lid and whisk in the corn, black beans, tempeh, pepper, and salt. Then again, cook for about 2-3 more minutes.

10. Spread cheddar cheese and bake till the cheese melts. (If you use the oven-safe skillet, you can also put it under the grill to melt the cheese at this level.)

11. Now you can do the seasoning with coriander, and present it.

Nutrition

- ✓ Calories 380
- ✓ Fat 18g
- ✓ Carbs 35g
- ✓ Protein 20g

Recipe 33: Poached Cod in a Tomato Broth

- o Total Time: 35 minutes
- o Serves: 4

Ingredients:

- Wild-caught cod fillet 1 pound
- Organic tomatoes (BPA-free), drained One 28-ounce can

- Pastured chicken stock 1.5 cups
- Small pinch of saffron
- Bay leaves 2
- Avocado oil three tablespoons
- Sea salt to taste

Instructions

1. Put oil in a frying pan that is set to medium heat.

2. Crush the sliced tomatoes into the oven with your fingertips. Attach to taste stock, saffron, leaves of the bay, and salt.

3. Bring broth over medium heat to boiling, then reducing heat to low.

4. Add cod fillets and put a cover on it, cook for 5-7 minutes till the fish begins to flake.

5. Serve the tomato broth dish.

Nutrition:

- ✓ Calories: 167
- ✓ Total Fat: 10.3g
- ✓ Carbs 8g
- ✓ Protein 27g

Recipe 34: Low Carb Cauliflower Bowl

- o Total Time: 25 minutes
- o Serves: 4

Ingredients

- Butter 3 tablespoons
- Diced onion ¼ cup
- Fresh cauliflower 2 cups

- Cream cheese, softened 2 ounces
- Pickled jalapeno slices one-fourth cup
- Brewed brisket 2 cups
- Shredded sharp cheddar 1 cup
- Diced green onions 2tbs.
- Cooked crumbled bacon one-fourth cup

- Heavy cream one-fourth cup

Instructions

1. Split the cauliflower into pieces of bite-size. Heat or cook till the pork gets tender and put it on one side.

2. Switch the moderate heat and put slices of onion, butter and jalapeno to the pot. Toast till you get the onions translucent.

3. Decrease heat gradually and add ready brisket or leftover beef or chicken along with cream cheese.

4. If the mixture is melting or burning too fast, decrease the flame of heat a little. Continue cooking till the cream cheese gets melted and mixed quickly.

5. Turn off the stroke.

6. Put sharp cheddar, heavy cream, and cauliflower.

7. Rapidly blend till the cheese is melted and merged.

8. Spread green onions, and crumbled bacon on the top surface. Serve hot.

Nutrition:

- ✓ Calories 329
- ✓ Carbs: 5g
- ✓ Protein: 18g
- ✓ Fat: 27g

Recipe 35: One Pan Roasted Chicken and Vegetables

Ingredients

- Bone-in thighs One and a half to two lbs.

- Cut into carrot sticks 12 oz.

- Whole carrots (6–8 medium)

- Baby red potatoes 12 oz.

- Green beans, washed and trimmed 12 oz.

- One big red onion, sliced into wedges

- Garlic cloves, minced 3-4

- Fresh thyme 2 tsp.

- Olive oil or avocado oil half tbsp.

- Sea salt and chili pepper half tsp.

Instructions

1. Settle the oven to 425 degrees F.

2. Put a large diameter, parchment-paper.

3. Toss on the baking sheet prepped and diced vegetables and herbs with butter.

4. Put the thighs of the chicken on the surface of the vegetables.

5. Season with salt and pepper as you like.

6. Bake for 30-35 minutes till chicken is cooked and potatoes soften. Throughout the preparation, shake and switch vegetables once or twice.

Nutrition:

- ✓ Calories 370
- ✓ Protein 26g

✓ Fat 16g
✓ Carbs 33g

Chapter 5: Snacks Recipes for Intermittent Fasting

When you are on Intermittent Fasting, you can enjoy your meals with different combos. As we are talking about 16:8 intermittent fasting diet regime, so, you have a lot of time to enjoy your favorite meals. In the previous chapters we discussed a bundle of recipes that you can choose according to your choice and the meal you are skipping and which you are taking as complementary meal. Whatever, meal plan you choose, you can relish the snacks. In this chapter, you are going to be provided with many delicious and easy to make snacks recipes. Keep reading to get more amazing recipes.

5.1 Easy to Make Snacks Recipes for Intermittent Fasting Protocol

Recipe 1: Chocolate Covered Almonds

o   Total Time: 15 minutes

o   Serves: 8

Ingredients

- Dark chocolate 400 grams
- Roasted whole almonds 1 cup

Instructions

1. Put parchment paper in a baking tray and keep it on one side.

2. Layer a baking sheet with parchment paper. Set aside.

3. Divide the dark chocolate into tiny chunks and place it in a heat-resistant container.

4. Position the chocolate bowl over the water pot. Ensure that the water does not hit the floor of the pot.

5. Put a pot of water to a boil.

6. Once the chocolate melts, take off from heat and mix till it is melted.

7. Combine and whisk till the almonds get fully coated with molten chocolate.

8. Take out one almond at a time two forks and put to the parchment layered baking sheet.

9. Separate as much chocolate as you can.

10. Then put in the refrigerator for some time and serve.

Nutrition

- ✓ Calories 170
- ✓ Carbs 7g

Recipe 2: Peach Smoothie

- o Total Time: 5 minutes
- o Serves: 1

Ingredients

- Peaches, frozen 1 cup
- Coconut milk one-fourth cup
- Almond flavor half tsp.
- Greek yogurt 1/2 cup

Instructions

1. Blend peaches, coconut milk, Greek yogurt, almond flavor in a high-speed mixer.

2. You can see the thickness and make it accordingly.

3. Finish with pretty toppings such as chia seeds, berries and almonds.

4. Enjoy it.

Nutrition

- ✓ Calories 150

Recipe 3: Broccoli Corn Bread

o Total Time: 45

o Serves: 12

Ingredients

- **Eggs (beaten)** 4
- Jiffy corn muffin mix 2 boxes
- Chopped broccoli (thawed and drained) 1 package
- Cottage cheese 1 cup
- Medium **onion** (chopped) 1
- **Melted butter_** one and a half stick

Instructions

1. Settle the oven at 375 F.

2. Apply the greasing of a medium baking pan.

3. Mix corn muffin mixes in a pot with melted butter, and beaten eggs.

4. Whisk in the washed broccoli, cottage cheese, and diced onion.

5. Put on the prepared baking tray.

6. Put for baking in the oven for about 35 to 40 minutes, or till slightly browned.

7. Present it!

Nutrition

- ✓ Calories 64
- ✓ Carbs 4g
- ✓ Fat 3g

✓ Protein 5g

Recipe 4: Mixed Sprouts Corn Chaat

- o Total Time: 30 minutes
- o Serves: 2

Ingredients

- Corn, boiled 15 g
- Mixed sprouts, boiled 15 g
- Onion, finely chopped 1
- Cumin powder 1/2 tsp
- Salt, to taste
- Coriander leaves, chopped Handful
- Red chili powder or paprika 1/2 tsp
- Tomato, finely chopped 1
- Coriander chutney 1 tbsp.
- Pomegranate seeds Handful

Instructions

1. Dip the sprouts overnight and cook the next morning pressure for around 10-15 minutes and strain.
2. Now in a bowl, mix all the ingredients and serve. It is simple to cook, quick to eat.

Nutrition

- ✓ Calorie 150
- ✓ Fat 1g
- ✓ Carbs 26.3g
- ✓ Protein 8.3g

Recipe 5: Chili Bowl

- o Total Time: 45 minutes
- o Serves: 6

Ingredients

- Extra-virgin olive oil 1 tbsp.

- Onion, chopped 1
- Fire-roasted diced tomatoes 15-oz.
- Chili powder 1 1/2 tbsp.
- Black beans, drained 15-oz.
- Kosher salt one-fourth tsp.
- Black pepper ¼ tsp.
- Tomato paste 2 tbsp.
- Ground beef 1 1/2 lb.
- Cloves of garlic, minced 3
- Low-sodium beef broth 2 c.
- Ground cumin 1 tsp.
- Kidney beans, drained 15-oz.
- Cayenne half tsp.
- Dried oregano 1 tsp.

Instructions

1. Cook onions for 5 minutes.
2. Put garlic and cook for 1 minute.
3. Add tomato paste and ground beef.
4. Cook for about seven minutes.
5. Add broth, beans, tomatoes, salt, pepper, chili powder, cumin, oregano, and cayenne.
6. Cook in pressure on high flame for 14 minutes.
7. Serve with desired toppings.

Nutrition

✓ Calories 310
✓ Carbs 28g

✓ Fat 10g

✓ Protein 30g

Recipe 6: Blueberry Cheese Cake Bars

- o Total Time 50 minutes

- o Serves 9

Ingredients

- Cream cheese 16 oz.

- Golden monk fruit sweetener 1/3 cup

- Pure vanilla extract One tsp.

- Eggs, beaten Three

- Tartar cream 1/4 tsp.

- Fresh blueberries 1 cup

- Baking soda 1/8 tsp.

Instructions

1. Settle the oven to 325 Fahrenheit and coat the baking pan with a sprinkle of non-stick cooking oil.

2. Then use an electric mixer, mix all ingredients in a mixing pot till fully incorporated, excluding blueberries.

3. Put the mixture into the baking pan prepared.

4. Put on top of the mixture blueberries.

5. Move the pan to the oven and bake for about 40-45 minutes until the crust is golden brown.

6. Take the pan from the oven after frying, cover the pan loosely with tape, and put the pan in the refrigerator for four hours.

7. Cut cheesecake into 12 bars of the same size with a knife, remove pan bars with a spatula, serve and enjoy!

Nutrition:

- ✓ Calorie 265
- ✓ Total Fat 13.2g
- ✓ Protein 4.3g
- ✓ Total Carbohydrate 8.6g

Recipe 7: Fudgy Keto Brownies

- o Total Time: 35 minutes
- o Serves: 16

Ingredients:

- Three eggs at room temperature
- Almond flour 1/2 cup
- Non-sweetened cocoa powder 1/4 cup
- Baking powder 1/2 cup
- Butter 12 cup
- Erythritol 3/4 cup
- Dark chocolate 2 oz.

Instructions

1. Settle the oven at 350 °F.
2. Make a layer with an 8-inch baking sheet of parchment paper that protects the bottom and the edges.
3. Mix the sugar with the dark chocolate in a tub. Microwave on a double boiler for 30 seconds or heat the mixture.

4. Meanwhile, whisk the dry ingredients: sweetener, almond flour, cocoa powder, and baking powder.

5. Blend the eggs in a bowl and put them with the mixer.

6. Add the mix of butter and chocolate and proceed to blend.

7. Mix in the dry ingredients slowly until you get the consistency of brownies powder.

8. Move the batter and bake for 15-20 minutes in the baking pan. The baking time varies for each oven.

9. Be sure you do not over bake them. On touching, the middle has to be somewhat wet.

10. Take the brownies from the oven and let them cool for about 10 minutes.

11. Cut your brownies into 16 pieces with a sharp knife and devour!

Nutrition

- ✓ Calories 135kcal
- ✓ Total Carbs 1.32g
- ✓ Protein 2g
- ✓ Fat 14g

Recipe 8: Peanut Butter Oatmeal Balls

- o Total Time: 20 minutes
- o Serves: 18 bites

Ingredients

- Shredded unsweetened coconut 1 cup
- Almond meal one-fourth cup
- Creamy peanut butter ¾ cup
- Old-fashioned oats gluten-free 1 cup
- Sea salt ¼ tsp

- Honey or maple syrup ¼ cup
- Unsweetened almond milk 2-4 tbs.
- Pure vanilla extract 1 tsp.

Instructions

1. Layer a baking sheet with parchment paper, put it aside.
2. In a large pot, combine old fashioned oats, almond meal, coconut, and salt. Put it on one side.
3. In a microwave-safe bowl or a saucepan over moderate heat, warm the peanut butter and honey till fine.
4. Take from heat and put 2 tbs. vanilla and almond milk
5. Put wet mixture to dry mix and whisk till completely combined.
6. Spoon out one tbs. of dough, make balls and put on prepared baking sheet.
7. Keep doing it, till all the dough used.
8. Put balls in the refrigerator or freezer to settle.
9. Change the bites from the baking sheet to an airtight box and put in the refrigerator.

Nutrition

- ✓ Calories 133
- ✓ Fat 9g
- ✓ Carbs 10g
- ✓ Protein 4.2g

Recipe 9: Honey Garlic Chicken Breasts

- o Total Time: 30 minutes
- o Serves: 4

Ingredients

- Low sodium soy sauce ¼ cup
- Honey one-fourth cup
- Water 1/3 cup

- Garlic, minced 2 cloves

- Black pepper one-fourth tsp

- Medium-size boneless skinless chicken breasts 1 1/2-pound

- Cornstarch 2 tsp.

Instructions

1. Combine water, soy sauce, honey, garlic, chicken, and pepper in Instant Pot.
2. Cook at High Pressure for 10 minutes.
3. In a bowl, mix 2 teaspoons cornstarch and 1 tablespoon water.
4. Cook cornstarch mixture on Sauté mode for 2-3 minutes.
5. Dip sliced chicken in sauce.
6. Serve with rice and vegetable.

Nutrition per serving

- ✓ Calories 323
- ✓ Fat 13g
- ✓ Carbs 23g
- ✓ Protein 28g

Recipe 10: Beet Hummus

- o Total Time: 1 hour 5 minutes

- o Serves: 16

Ingredients

- Beets, peeled and quartered 2 large

- Lemon juice one-fourth cup

- Olive oil and more for roasting beets 32g

- Chickpeas 2 cups

- Kosher salt, divided 1/2 tsp.

- Water 1/3 cup
- Tahini 2 tbsp.
- Garlic, grated 1 clove

Instructions

1. Settle your oven to 375°F.
2. Coat beets with olive oil and wrap beets in aluminium foil,
3. Roast in the oven while baking sheet for 40 to 60 minutes.
4. Place half cup dried chickpeas and water in the Instant Pot.
5. Cook for 40 minutes on high pressure.
6. Reserve chickpea cooking liquid.
7. Place roasted beets, chickpeas, lemon juice, tahini and salt in the food processor.
8. Blend until nearly smooth.
9. Add in olive oil while the food processor is running.
10. Add in water or reserved cooking liquid from chickpeas to get the hummus creamy and serve.

Nutrition

- ✓ Calories 165
- ✓ Carbs 7g
- ✓ Fat 14g
- ✓ Protein 3g

Recipe 11: Lemon Curd

- o Total Time: 5 minutes
- o Serves 3

Ingredients:

- Lemons (Juice and Zest) 4
- Natvia 1/2 cup
- Butter 100 g
- Whole Eggs 3
- Egg Yolk 1

Instructions

1. Squeeze the lemons and add zest.
2. Put Natvia and put butter to a medium heat-proof bowl.
3. Place the container over a water pan that is softly boiling. Do not let the bowl hit the pan's edge. Stir the mixture until the butter has cooled.
4. Whisk the yolk of the egg gently, then whisk in the warm mixture. Stir and simmer until the paste covers the back of a spoon for about 10 minutes.
5. Remove from heat and put the mixture in sterilized jars and store for up to 2 weeks in the refrigerator.

Nutrition

- ✓ Calories 258kcal
- ✓ Fat 25g
- ✓ Protein 7g
- ✓ Carbs 2g

Recipe 12: Peanut Butter Jelly Apple Nachos

- o Total Time 5 minutes
- o Serves 1

Ingredients

- Jelly, your favorite flavor 1-2 tablespoons
- Large apple 1
- Smooth peanut butter, melted 1-2 tablespoons
- Chia seeds, optional

Instructions

1. Dice apple thinly into slices and put on a plate.
2. Make a topping with jelly and melted peanut butter
3. You can top with a seasoning of chia seeds or nuts.
4. Enjoy!

Nutrition

- ✓ Calories 265
- ✓ Total fat 6g
- ✓ Carbohydrates 50g
- ✓ Protein 5g

Recipe 13: Pumpkin Cake Pops

- o Total Time: 15 minutes
- o Serves: 12

Ingredients

- **Coconut flour** sifted 1 cup
- **Pumpkin puree** not pumpkin pie filling 1/2-3/4 cup
- **Granulated sweetener of choice** 1/4 cup
- **Dairy free chocolate chips** optional 1/4 cup
- Cinnamon to taste optional

Instructions

1. Settle the oven to 350 and oil a baking tray and put it on one side.

2. Take a large mixing bowl, mix the pumpkin puree, coconut flour, cinnamon, and granulated sweetener.
3. If you use chocolate chips, whisk them till fully incorporated.
4. With your hands, form small balls and put on the greased sheet.
5. According to your desired texture bake, for about ten minutes (for a soft texture of cake) or for 15 minutes (crumbly and dense texture).
6. Take from oven and cool completely before eating.

Nutrition

- ✓ Calories 219
- ✓ Carbs 322g
- ✓ Fat 43g
- ✓ Protein 23g

Recipe 14: Baked Veggie Chips

- o Total Time 25 minutes
- o Serves 4

Ingredients

- Carrot 1 large
- Golden Beetroot 1 medium
- Zucchini 1 medium
- Beetroot 1 medium
- Small Sweet Potato 1
- Pepper Adjust to taste 1/2 tsp
- Small turnip 1
- Sea salt Adjust to taste 1/2 tsp
- Oil Optional 1 spritz

Instructions

1. Set the oven to 400F.
2. Cut all the veggies into thin pieces with a knife.

3.   In a bowl, mix these veggies with salt, oil and pepper till evenly coated.
4.   Scatter on baking pan layered with parchment paper.
5.   Set to bake for 10 minutes at 400F. and change sides.
6.   Bake for more 5-10 minutes till crispy and lightly brown.
7.   Take out from the oven and cool for some minutes before eating.

Nutrition

- ✓ Calories 195
- ✓ Fat 9.6g
- ✓ Carbs 24g
- ✓ Protein 5g

Recipe 15: Mediterranean Pinwheels

- o Total Time: 6minutes
- o Serves: 16

Ingredients

- Tahini Paste 3 tbs.
- Lemon juice 3 tbs.
- Garlic 1 clove
- White vinegar 4 tbs.
- Water half cup
- Pepper and salt to taste
- For Making Pinwheels
- Cherry tomatoes
- Olives
- Lettuce
- Artichokes in a jar
- Tortillas, gluten-free
-

Instructions

Tahini Sauce

1. Mix all ingredients in a pot till you get a smooth paste.

For Pinwheels

1. Chop tomatoes, olives, and artichokes, into pieces.
2. Apply one tbs. of the Tahini sauce over one tortilla.
3. Put vegetables and add with a handful of salads.
4. Firmly roll the tortillas and cut in shape of pinwheels.

Nutrition

- ✓ Calories 190
- ✓ Carbs 14.2g
- ✓ Fat 12.6g
- ✓ Protein 5.6g

Recipe 16: Chocolate Coconut Smoothie (Especially for Athletes)

- o Total Time: 15 minutes
- o Serves: 1

Ingredients:

- Full-fat tin organic coconut milk 0.25 cup
- Liquid coconut stevia 15-20 drops
- Unsweetened raw cacao powder 2 tablespoon
- Ice (just enough to thicken)
- Collagen protein   2 scoops

Instructions

1. Put all the components in a mixer, but not collagen, and mix.

2. Put collagen and shake to combine.

3. Put in a mug and add garnishes.

4. Serve instantly, or put in fridge.

Nutrition

- ✓ Calories: 500kcal
- ✓ Protein: 26g
- ✓ Total Carbs: 12g
- ✓ Fat: 38g

Recipe 17: Low Carb Cucumber Green Tea Detox Smoothie

- o Total Time: 5 minutes
- o Serves: 2

Ingredients:

- Water 8 ounces

- Green tea powder 2 tsp.

- Sliced cucumber 1 cup

- Ripe avocado 2 ounces

- Lemon juice 1 tsp.

- Stevia liquid lemon 1/2 tsp.

- Ice 1/2 cup

Instructions

1. Put water and green tea powder into a mixer and mix with a whirl.

2. Put the other ingredients and mix well until smooth.

3. Sweetener to taste and change as needed.

4. Serve or refrigerate till you are ready to serve.

Nutrition

✓ Calories 69

✓ Net Carbs: 3.4g

✓ Fat 4.6g

✓ Fibber 3.4g

✓ Protein 2g

Recipe 18: Fish Cakes

- o Total Time: 30 minutes
- o Serves: 16 fish cakes

Ingredients

- Raw white boneless fish 1 pound
- Cilantro 1/4 cup
- Pinch of salt
- Chili flakes Pinch
- Garlic cloves (optional) 1-2
- Coconut oil 1 -2 tablespoons
- Avocado oil

Dipping Sauce:

- Lemon, juiced 1
- Ripe avocados 2
- Salt one pinch
- Water 2tablespoons

Instructions

1. Put vegetables, rice, garlic, chili, butter and pork in a food processor. Whisk till all is mixed.

2. Put coconut oil in a large pan over moderate heat.

3. Shape the mixture of fish into six patties.

4. In the hot pan, incorporate cookies. Continue cooking unless golden brown on both sides and cook evenly.

5. When cooking fish cakes, put to a small food processor or blender and blitz all dipping sauce ingredients till smooth and creamy.

6. Taste the mixture and, if necessary, put more lemon juice or salt.

7. Serve warm with dipping sauce when the fish cakes get ready. It is a serving of six individuals.

Nutrition

- ✓ Calories 69
- ✓ Protein 1.1g
- ✓ Total Fat 6.5g
- ✓ Total Carbs 2.7g

Recipe 19: Chicken Wings

- o Total Time: 50 minutes
- o Serves: 8

Ingredients

- Chicken wings 4 lb.
- Garlic powder 1 tsp.
- Paprika 1 tsp.
- Kosher salt 1 tsp.
- Freshly ground black pepper 1 tsp.
- Hot sauce half c.
- Butter half c.

Instructions

1. Layer 2 medium-size baking sheets with aluminum foil.
2. Combine chicken wings with garlic powder, salt, paprika, and pepper.
3. Add water and wings on trivet.
4. High-Pressure Cook 10 minutes.
5. In a microwave-safe bowl, melt butter.
6. Add butter in hot sauce.
7. Toss wings with 1/2 the sauce.
8. Adjust in an even layer on the prepared baking sheet and broil for 4 minutes per side.
9. Gently toss with remaining sauce and serve.

Nutritional Value

✓ Calories 290
✓ Fat 17g
✓ Carbs 14g
✓ Protein 19g

Recipe 20: Grape and Melon Juice

o Serves: 1
o Total Time: 2 minutes

Ingredients

- Cucumber, peeled ½
- Red grapes seedless 100g
- Baby spinach leaves 30g
- Cantaloupe melon, peeled, deseeded 100g

Instructions

1. Mix all the ingredients in a juicer or blender until smooth and it is ready to serve.

Nutrition

- ✓ Calories 97
- ✓ Carb 12g
- ✓ Protein 4g
- ✓ Fat 3g

Recipe 21: Matcha Green Tea

- o Total Time: 5 minutes
- o Serves: 1

Ingredients

- Ice 1 cup
- Matcha powder 2 teaspoons
- Cold vanilla almond milk 2-3 ounces
- Cold water 1/2 cup
- A little bit of vanilla

Instructions

- o Put ice into a bottle and put two teaspoons of matcha powder.
- o Apply half a cup of cold water, stir the mixture well and put in an ice-filled bottle.
- o For preparing this latte, we put 2-3 oz. of cold, vanilla almond milk into the glass and sometimes whisk in a splash of coffee.
- o Calories: 20

Recipe 22: Potato Salad

- o Total Time: 26 minutes
- o Serve: 5

Ingredients

- Russet potatoes 3 lbs.
- Eggs 3

- Mustard 2 tsp.
- Salt half tsp.
- Black pepper one-fourth tsp.
- Water 1.5 cups
- Mayo 1.5 cup
- Sour cream one-fourth cup

Instructions

1. Chop peeled potatoes into ½ inch cubes.
2. Add to the Instant Pot and put eggs on top.
3. Add water.
4. Cook at High Pressure for 4 minutes.
5. Chop eggs and mix with potatoes.
6. Add mayo, sour cream, mustard and salt, and pepper.
7. Chill for 1 hour and serve.

Nutrition

- ✓ Calories 300
- ✓ Carbs 50

Recipe 23: Berries Smoothie

- o Total Time: 5 minutes
- o Serves: 2

Ingredients

- Frozen strawberries half cup
- Almond milk half cup
- Frozen blueberries half cup
- Agave nectar 1tsp.
- Flaxseed oil 1tsp.
- Low fat Yogurt half cup

Instructions

Mix almond milk, blueberries, strawberries, flax seed oil, yogurt, and agave nectar in a mixer till smooth.

Nutrition

- ✓ Calorie 230
- ✓ Fat 5.3g
- ✓ Carbs 7.4mg
- ✓ Protein 8.7g

Recipe 24: Cobb Salad Dip

- o Total Time: 30 minutes
- o Serves: 4

Ingredients

- Sour cream 1 cup
- Light cream cheese, softened 8 ounces
- Chopped Romaine lettuce 1 cup
- Shredded cheddar cheese ½ cup
- Bacon, cooked & crumbled 2 strips
- Chopped Roma tomato 1 cup
- Corn ½ cup
- Ranch mix 2 tablespoons
- Blue cheese crumbles ¼ cup
- Blue corn/corn tortillas to serve

Instructions

1. Take a normal size pot, and mix sour cream, cream cheese, and ranch seasoning till smooth.
2. Make a layer with it at the bottom of a nine-inch plate.

3. Put salad, cheddar cheese, chopped tomatoes corn, blue cheese, and bacon

4. You can enjoy with tortillas.

Nutrition

- ✓ Calories 70
- ✓ Fat 6g
- ✓ Carbs 2g
- ✓ Protein 2g

Recipe 25: Peanut Butter Chocolate Dip

- o Total Time: 5 minutes
- o Serves: 2

Ingredients

- Vanilla yogurt 6 ounces

- Peanut butter 1 tablespoon

- Unsweetened Cocoa powder 2 tablespoons

- Apple slices, Strawberries, and other fruit

- Maple syrup or honey 1 tablespoon

Instructions

1. Take a normal size bowl, mix all ingredients.

2. Put in refrigerator for about 30 minutes and it is ready.

Nutrition

- ✓ Calories 30
- ✓ Fat 0.6g
- ✓ Carbs 2.8g
- ✓ Protein 4g

Recipe 26: Guacamole Bar

- o Total Time: 10 minutes
- o Serves: 6

Ingredients

- Serrano or other fresh green chilies, finely chopped 1-2
- Red onion, very finely chopped 1/2
- Ripe Hass avocados 3
- Sea salt 1-2 tsp
- Limes Juice 1-2
- Black pepper
- Coriander leaves, chopped

Instructions

1. Make paste of a quarter of onion and half chili and salt in a pestle and mortar.

2. Cut avocados, take out the stones and spoon out the flesh into the mortar.

3. Mash the pulp with a fork, add half of lime juice.

4. Once you have a rough guacamole, mix in the leftover lime juice, chili, red onion and coriander.

5. Sprinkle pinch of black pepper and some salt.

6. Present with tortilla chips.

Nutrition

- ✓ Calories 109
- ✓ Fat 10g
- ✓ Carbs 6g

Recipe 27: Strawberry Banana Pancake

- o Total Time: 15 minutes

- o Serves 4

Ingredients

- Bananas
- Strawberries
- Flour 1 cup
- Baking powder 2 tablespoons
- Egg 1
- Sugar 2 tablespoons
- Pinch of salt
- Milk one and a half cup
- Butter, melted 1 tablespoon
- Powdered sugar, and maple syrup, if you want

Instructions

1. Take a broad bowl for combining dry ingredients.
2. Beat milk, egg, and butter in another utensil. Then mix with dry ingredients.
3. Stir the mixture just enough to moisten the flour.
4. Shift the dough into a big bottle take you can use for squeezing.
5. Take a pan that is not sticky, put a quarter amount of material
6. Turn when bubbles start rising and the bottom becomes brown.
7. Once the pancakes are ready, assemble from lower part to top like a pancake, banana, and strawberry.
8. Do it one more time to finish with a pancake at the upper side.

9. You can top with maple syrup, and powdered sugar.

Nutrition

- ✓ Calories 89.7
- ✓ Carbs 18g
- ✓ Fat 0.6g
- ✓ Protein 3.2g

Recipe 28: Mango Turmeric Smoothie Bowl

- o Total Time:15 minutes
- o Serves: 1 bowl

Ingredients

- Black berries
- Lime zest
- Toasted slivered almonds
- Goji berries
- Cereal or granola
- Coconut flakes
- Chia seeds or flax seeds

Instructions

1. Put mango slices and banana to a food processing machine.
2. Thaw the fruit for 5-10 minutes.
3. Put almond milk, vanilla extract, turmeric, lime juice, coconut extract.
4. Mix till smooth and no pieces are there.
5. Shift to a bowl and garnish with toppings.

Nutrition

- ✓ Calorie 226

Recipe 29: Wheat Berry Salad

- o Total Time: 40 minutes
- o Serves: 6

Ingredients

- Wheat berries 1 cup
- Olive oil, divided 3 tbsp.
- Orange juice 1/4 cup
- Salt 1/2 tsp.
- Balsamic vinegar 1 tbsp.
- Water, divided 2 1/4 cups
- Apples, diced 2
- Shredded carrots 2 cups
- Raisins 1/2 cup
- Orange zest 2 tsp.
- Pure maple syrup 2 tbsp.

Instructions

1. Sauté wheat berries in oil for 4–5 minutes.

2. Cook at Manual for 30 minutes.

3. Transfer cooled berries to a bowl.

4. Add remaining ingredients.

5. Refrigerate and serve.

Nutrition

- ✓ Calories 190
- ✓ No saturated fat
- ✓ Protein 6gm
- ✓ Carbs 15g

Recipe 30: Bulletproof Coffee

- o Total Time: 2 minutes
- o Serves: 1

Ingredients

- Brewed coffee 8 to 12 ounces
- Brain octane oil1 tablespoon
- Grass-fed, unsalted butter 1 tablespoon

Instructions

1. Prepare one cup of coffee with pure water with coffee brewer.

2. Put this coffee in a blender. Then add one tbsp. of Brain Octane and 1 tbsp. of grass-fed butter.

3. Mix for about 30 seconds till the coffee looks as a foamy latte.

4. Put it in a mug and savor each sip.

Nutrition

- ✓ Calories 226
- ✓ Fat 25g
- ✓ Carbs 0
- ✓ Protein o.5g

Recipe 31: Spaghetti

- o Total Time: 30 minutes
- o Serves: 5

Ingredients:

- Dried Italian seasoning 1 tsp.

- Lean ground turkey 1-pound

- Regular uncooked spaghetti 8 oz.

- Jar marinara sauce 25-ounce

- Garlic powder ½ tsp.

- Salt ½ tsp.

- Black pepper one-fourth tsp.

- Water 2 cups

Instructions

1. Turn Instant Pot to Sauté mode.

2. Cook ground turkey until browned and remove.

3. Mix Italian seasoning, garlic powder, salt, pepper, and water.

4. Add the halved spaghetti noodles.

5. Pour marinara sauce over the spaghetti.

6. Cook at High Pressure for 7 minutes.

7. Let cool for 3-5 minutes and then serve.

Nutrition

- ✓ Total Calories 200
- ✓ Carbs 40g
- ✓ Fat 1.3g
- ✓ Protein 8.2g

Recipe 32: Bone Broth

- o Total Time: 40 minutes
- o Serves: 4

Ingredients

- Carcass of chicken along with roasted juice 1
- Garlic clove 1
- Lemon juice and zest 1
- Ground coriander 1 tsp

- Bay leaves 2
- Red chilies, halved, deseeded and sliced 1-2
- Ground cumin ½ tsp
- Coriander, leaves chopped

Instructions

1. Put chicken carcass in a pan.

2. Put onion, one and a half liter of water, bay leaves, and the lemon juice.

3. Put a cover and cook for about 40 minutes.

4. Take it off from the stove and let it cool.

5. Put a strainer on a pot and separate all the bones from the liquid.

6. Make strips of chicken.

7. Put all the broth from the pot to the pan along with roasting juices.

8. Put ground coriander, chili, cumin, lemon zest, coriander stems and garlic.

9. Cook for some more minutes till bubbling.

10. Check the texture.

Nutrition

- ✓ Calories 150
- ✓ Protein 6g
- ✓ Fat 3g
- ✓ Carbs 24g

Recipe 33: Green Bean and Tomato Salad

- o Total Time: 25 minutes
- o Serves: 2

Ingredients

- Chopped cilantro 1/4 cup
- Basil, chopped 2 tbsp.
- Chopped roasted cashews 2 tbsp.
- Green beans, cut into 1-inch pieces 6 oz.
- Kosher salt 1/4 tsp.
- Cherry tomatoes, halved 3/4 cup

For the Dressing

- Garlic clove, minced 1
- lime juice 2 tsp.
- Fresh red chili chopped
- Fish sauce 2 tsp.
- Sugar 2 tsp.

Instructions

1. Put green beans in a steamer basket.

2. Add water and basket to the Pot.

3. Cook at High Pressure for 10 minutes.

4. Mix all ingredients for the dressing.

5. Sprinkle beans with salt and let cool.

6. Add the beans, cilantro, basil, cashews, and tomatoes to the dressing and serve.

Nutrition

- ✓ Calories 127
- ✓ Fat 4.9g
- ✓ Carbs 16.9g
- ✓ Protein 7.1g

Recipe 34: Boiled Eggs with Mayonnaise

- o Total Time: 10 minutes
- o Serves: 2

Ingredients

- Two eggs
- Two tablespoons of mayonnaise
- Two avocados

Instructions

1. Take water in a kettle to a boil.
2. Place the eggs in the water with care.
3. For soft-boiled eggs, boil the eggs for 5–6 minutes, for medium 6–8 minutes and for hard-boiled eggs for 8–10 minutes.
4. Serve with mayonnaise and chopped avocados.

Nutrition

- ✓ Calories 616
- ✓ Carbs 1 g
- ✓ Fat 84 g
- ✓ Protein 11 g

Conclusion

16:8 intermittent fasting includes feasting in an 8-hour duration and fasting for 16 hours. It supports weight loss and improves blood sugar, brain function, and longevity. You can enjoy healthy eating during your feasting time and have calorie-free drinks like water, herbal teas, and coffee. More than 100 recipes have been mentioned in the above chapters comprising of different meals that you can make from veggies, meat, fish, fruits, whole grains, and nuts. You can easily make different variations in your 16:8 fasting plan by adopting the protocols described in earlier chapters. Delicious recipes of breakfast, brunch, lunch, snacks, and dinner have been added to fulfill your selected type of fasting times and delicious eating experience. Intermittent Fasting Cookbook has been designed with an aim to provide you with the tastiest and most unique recipes ever.